73

SMP 11-16

Book B

D1148789

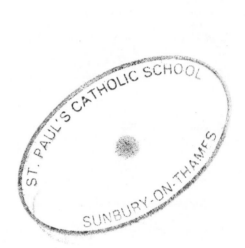
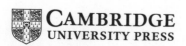

CAMBRIDGE
UNIVERSITY PRESS

PUBLISHED BY THE PRESS SYNDICATE OF THE UNIVERSITY OF CAMBRIDGE
The Pitt Building, Trumpington Street, Cambridge CB2 1RP, United Kingdom

CAMBRIDGE UNIVERSITY PRESS
The Edinburgh Building, Cambridge CB2 2RU, United Kingdom
40 West 20th Street, New York, NY 10011–4211, USA
10 Stamford Road, Oakleigh, Melbourne 3166, Australia

First published 1985
Eleventh printing 1996

Printed in the United Kingdom at the University Press, Cambridge

Set in MPlantin

A catalogue record for this book is available from the British Library

Library of Congress Cataloguing in Publication data

School Mathematics Project.
    SMP 11–16 blue series.
    Bk B1
    1. Mathematics – 1961–
    I. Title
    510   QA39.2

ISBN 0 521 31753 3 Paperback

Contents

1 Area (1)

A Calculating areas

Small areas can be measured in square centimetres.

The short way of writing 'square centimetres' is **cm²**.

The area of the rectangle on the right is 12 cm².

We can work out the area in cm² by multiplying the length in cm by the height in cm.

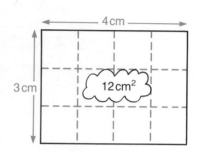

Larger areas can be measured in square metres (**m²**).

Here is the plan of a large room. Each small square on the plan stands for a square 1 metre by 1 metre.

We can work out the area of the room by splitting it into two rectangles.

Rectangle A is 8 m by 5 m, so its area is $8 \times 5 = 40 \, \text{m}^2$.

Rectangle B is 12 m by 4 m, so its area is $12 \times 4 = 48 \, \text{m}^2$.

So the total area of the room is

$$40 \, \text{m}^2 + 48 \, \text{m}^2 = \mathbf{88 \, m^2}.$$

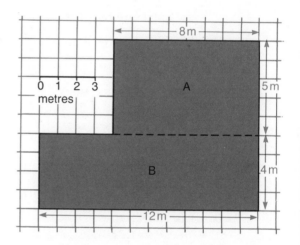

A1 Here is a different way of splitting up the area of the room.

(a) Calculate area C.

(b) Calculate area D.

(c) Check that the total area is the same as before.

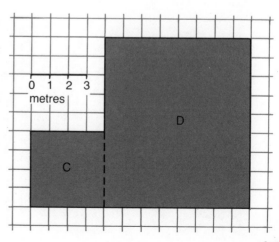

1

A2 Here are two different ways of splitting up the same floor area into rectangles.

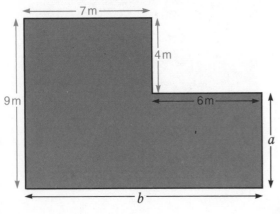

(a) Calculate the areas A and B, and add them together.

(b) Calculate the areas C, D and E, and add them together.

A3 This is a plan of a garden.

(a) Calculate the length marked a.

(b) Calculate the length marked b.

(c) Sketch the plan. Split the garden into two rectangles and work out the area of the garden.

A4 This is the floor plan of a house.

The widths marked w are both equal.

(a) Work out w.

(b) Calculate the total area of the floor.

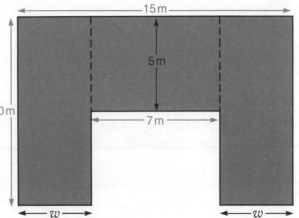

A5 Make a rough sketch of each of these shapes.
Work out the lengths marked with letters.
Calculate the area of each shape, in m².

(a)

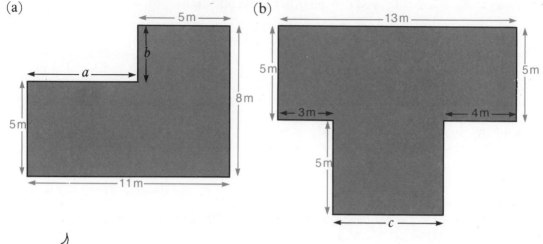

(b)

A6 If a house is destroyed by fire, the cost of rebuilding it is about £500 for every square metre of floor area.

If the house has two floors, their areas have to be added together.

The floor plans of this house are shown below.

(a) Calculate the area of the ground floor.

(b) Calculate the area of the first floor.

(c) Calculate the total cost of rebuilding the house after a fire.

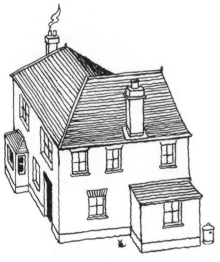

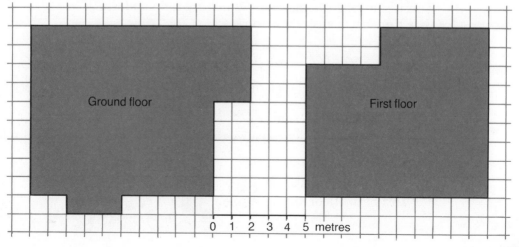

3

B Further multiplications

You know that $3 \times 2 = 6$.
Starting from $3 \times 2 = 6$, you can get other multiplications.

For example, if you change the 3 to 30, then the 6 becomes 60.

The pattern is shown in this diagram.

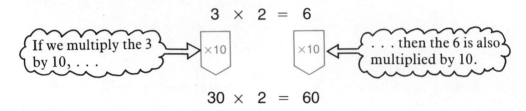

$$3 \times 2 = 6$$

If we multiply the 3 by 10, . . . ×10   ×10 . . . then the 6 is also multiplied by 10.

$$30 \times 2 = 60$$

Now the pattern can be continued.
Starting from $30 \times 2 = 60$, we can change the 2 to 20, like this.

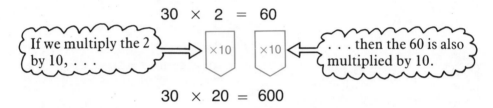

$$30 \times 2 = 60$$

If we multiply the 2 by 10, . . . ×10 ×10 . . . then the 60 is also multiplied by 10.

$$30 \times 20 = 600$$

B1 Use the answer to 4×7 to write down the answers to

(a) 4×70 (b) 40×7 (c) 40×70

B2 Work these out without using a calculator.

(a) 50×30 (b) 40×50 (c) 60×30 (d) 50×50

(e) 60×40 (f) 20×20 (g) 50×60 (h) 8×30

B3 This is someone's homework. Which are right and which wrong?
Give the correct answers to those which are wrong.

(a) $40 \times 40 = 160$ (b) $30 \times 70 = 2100$ (c) $80 \times 4 = 3200$
(d) $30 \times 30 = 60$ (e) $50 \times 20 = 1000$ (f) $60 \times 60 = 1200$
(g) $20 \times 20 = 40$ (h) $20 \times 40 = 800$ (i) $70 \times 70 = 490$

B4 Work out the area of this
rectangle without using
a calculator.

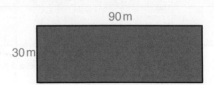

90 m

30 m

Look carefully at the pattern here.

Every time one of the numbers on the left of the = sign is multiplied by 10, the answer is also multiplied by 10.

Starting from $2 \times 4 = 8$, we can get the answer to 20×400.

$$2 \times 4 = 8$$
$$20 \times 4 = 80$$
$$20 \times 40 = 800$$
$$20 \times 400 = 8000$$

B5 (a) Starting from $3 \times 6 = 18$, work out 300×60.

(b) Starting from $4 \times 5 = 20$, work out 40×500.

(c) Starting from $3 \times 3 = 9$, work out 300×300.

B6 Work out (a) 20×300 (b) 300×40 (c) 50×200 (d) 100×100

B7 There are 60 seconds in a minute and 60 minutes in an hour. How many seconds are there in an hour?

B8 Without using a calculator, work out the lengths marked with letters in these diagrams, and the area of each shape.

Do not mark the page. Sketch the diagrams if you want to.

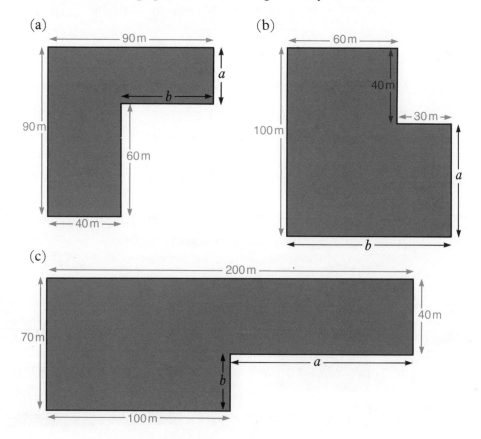

(a)

(b)

(c)

C Squares

A square is a rectangle whose sides are all the same length.

We work out the area of a square by multiplying the length of
a side by itself.

This diagram shows the areas of squares of side 1 cm, 2 cm, 3 cm and 4 cm.

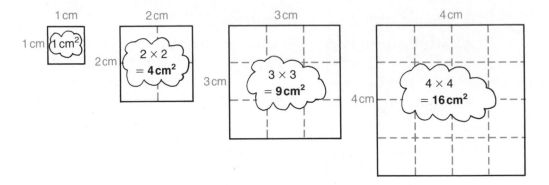

C1 (a) Copy and complete this table, to show the areas of squares
of side 1 cm, 2 cm, 3 cm, and so on up to 10 cm.

Length of side of square, in cm	1	2	3	4	5	6	7	8	9	10
Area of square, in cm²	1	4	9	16						

(b) The numbers in the bottom row of the table are called
square numbers.
What is the next square number, after 100?

(c) What is the next square number, after that?

C2 Without using a calculator, work out the area of each of
these squares. All measurements are in metres.

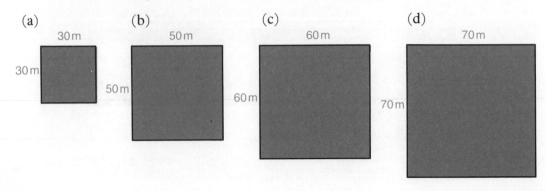

*D Calculating areas by subtraction

This is a plan of a garden.

There is a rectangular flower bed in the garden. The rest of the garden is grass (shaded).

We can calculate the area of the grass by **subtracting** the area of the flower bed from the total area of the garden.

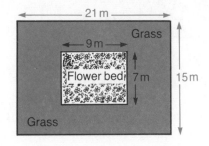

D1 (a) Calculate the total area of the whole garden.

   (b) Calculate the area of the flower bed.

   (c) Calculate the area of the grass.

   (d) The grass area has to be re-seeded. One kilogram of grass seed will cover about $25 \, m^2$.
   Roughly how much grass seed will be needed?

D2 Calculate the shaded area in each of these diagrams.

   Set out each calculation like this: Total area   = . . .

   Area of pond
   (or whatever) = . . .

   Shaded area   = . . .

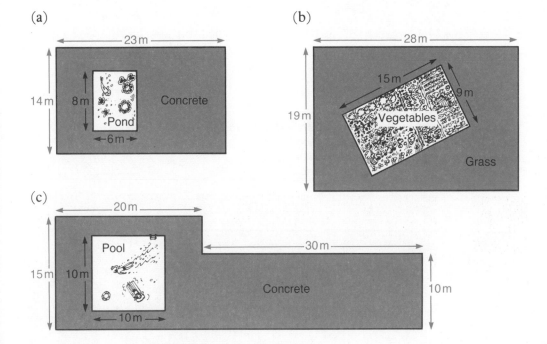

(a)

(b)

(c)

2 Patterns (1)

A Reflection symmetry

Each of these designs has a **line of reflection symmetry**.
If you stand a mirror on the line of symmetry, the design looks the same.

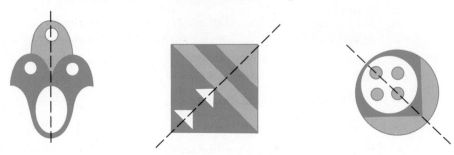

A1 Which of these designs have a line of reflection symmetry?

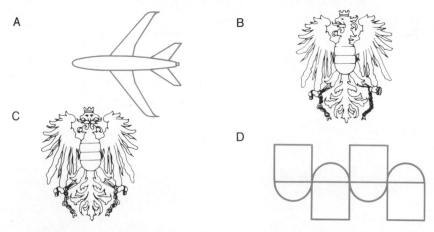

A

B

C

D

A2 Copy these drawings on squared paper.
Complete each drawing so that the dotted line is a line of
reflection symmetry.

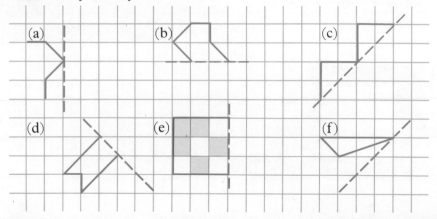

(a)   (b)   (c)

(d)   (e)   (f)

This design has 3 lines of reflection symmetry.

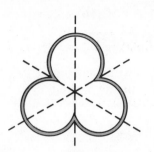

A3 How many lines of reflection symmetry does each of these shapes have? Draw sketches to show where the lines are.

Be careful! One of the shapes has no line of symmetry.

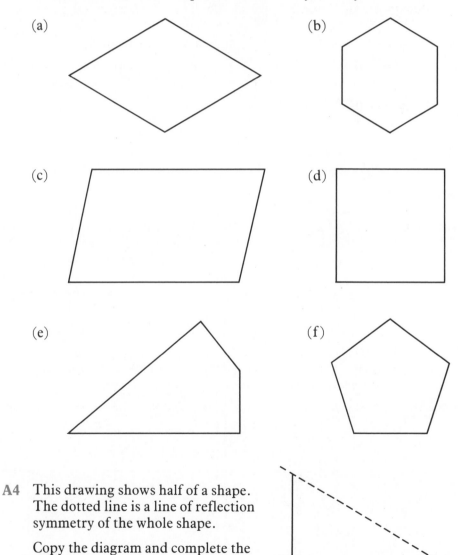

(a)

(b)

(c)

(d)

(e)

(f)

A4 This drawing shows half of a shape. The dotted line is a line of reflection symmetry of the whole shape.

Copy the diagram and complete the shape.

B 2-fold rotation centres

You need tracing paper.

None of these designs has a line of reflection symmetry.
(If you think any of them does have a line of symmetry, put a mirror
on them and see what happens.)

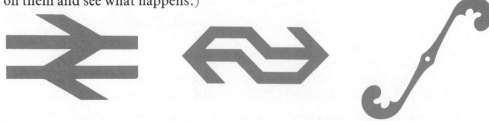
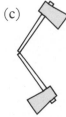

Ask someone to turn this page in his or her book upside down. Now compare
the upside-down page with the right-way-up page.
Each design looks exactly the same when it is turned upside down.

B1 Which of these designs look exactly the same upside down?
Try to answer this question without turning the page upside down.

(a) (b) (c)

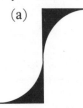
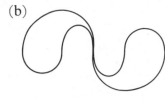
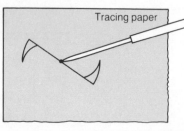

1 Trace this design.

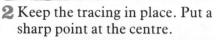

2 Keep the tracing in place. Put a
sharp point at the centre.

Tracing paper

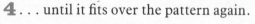

3 Rotate the tracing . . .

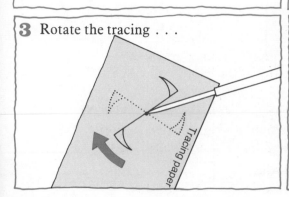

Tracing paper

4 . . . until it fits over the pattern again.

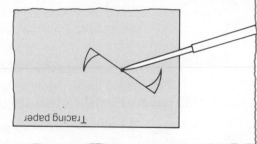

Tracing paper

There are 2 positions where the tracing fits over the pattern.

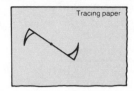
Tracing paper

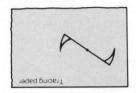
Tracing paper.

The centre where you put the sharp point is called the **2-fold rotation centre**, because there are 2 positions where the tracing fits.

(The word 'fold' here has nothing to do with folding paper.)

A special symbol is used to show a 2-fold rotation centre.
It looks like this: ➖

B2   *You need worksheet B1 – 1 (top half).*

Do this for each design on the worksheet.

(1) Trace the design.

(2) Keep the tracing in place. Put a sharp point through the dot on the design and rotate the tracing. See if there is one other position where the tracing fits over the design.

(3) If there is one other position, the design has a 2-fold rotation centre. Write 'yes' on the line under the design. Otherwise write 'no'.

B3   *You need worksheet B1 – 1 (bottom half).*

This is the Greek alphabet. It is printed on the worksheet.

ΑΒΓΔΕΖΗΘΙΚΛΜΝ
ΞΟΠΡΣΤΥΦΧΨΩ

(a) Trace the letter Θ (called 'theta') on the worksheet.
Put a sharp point at the centre of the letter.
Rotate your tracing until it fits again.
Mark the 2-fold rotation centre on the worksheet, using ➖ .

(b) There are eight more letters with 2-fold rotation centres. Trace them and mark their 2-fold rotation centres on the worksheet.

B4 Which of the cards below have a 2-fold rotation centre?
Do not trace the cards or turn the page upside down.
Imagine yourself rotating each card, and ask yourself: Will it
look exactly the same upside down?

A

B

C

D

E

F

B5 Which of these number plates have a 2-fold rotation centre?

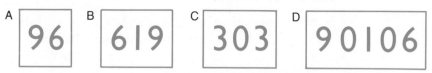

A 96   B 619   C 303   D 90106

B6 Copy these diagrams on squared paper.
Complete each one so that the point marked C is a
2-fold rotation centre. Check by tracing and turning.

(The first one has been done as an example.)

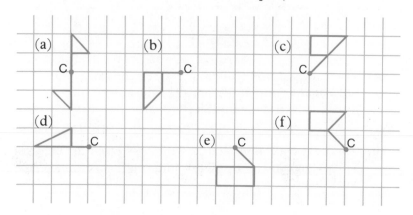

(a)   (b)   (c)   (d)   (e)   (f)

You need triangular spotty paper and tracing paper.

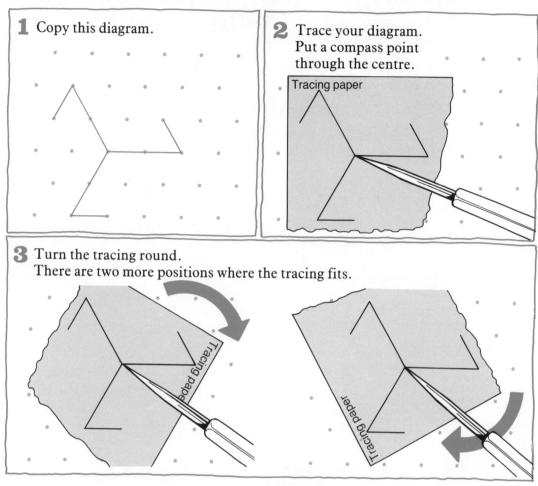

1 Copy this diagram.

2 Trace your diagram.
Put a compass point
through the centre.

Tracing paper

3 Turn the tracing round.
There are two more positions where the tracing fits.

Tracing paper

Tracing paper

Altogether there are **3 positions** where the tracing fits over the diagram.
The centre of the diagram is a **3-fold rotation centre**.

C1 Which of these diagrams have 3-fold rotation centres?
Use tracing paper to help, if you like.

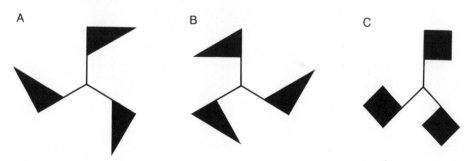

A

B

C

13

C2 Copy these diagrams.
Make each one into a diagram with a 3-fold rotation centre at the point C.

The first one is done as an example. You can check your answers by tracing and rotating.

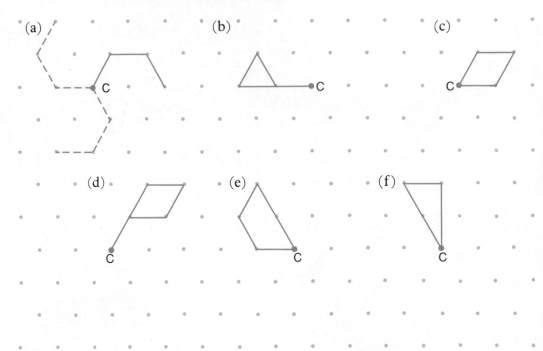

(a)　(b)　(c)

(d)　(e)　(f)

This design has a **4-fold rotation centre**.

If you trace the design and rotate the tracing about the centre, there are 4 positions where the tracing fits over the design.

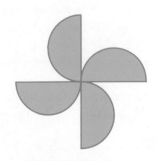

C3 Copy each of these diagrams on squared paper.
Make each one into a pattern with a 4-fold rotation centre at C.

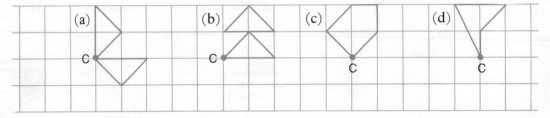

(a)　(b)　(c)　(d)

3 Rounding

A Rounding off large numbers

Blagdon Town football team have just had their worst defeat ever.

The newspaper headline gives the size of the crowd as 4700, but the exact number was 4683.

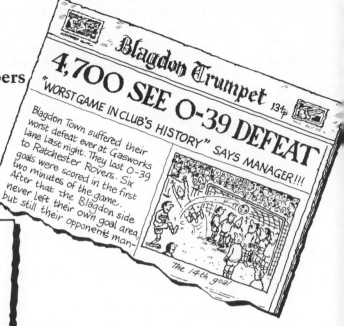

Gordian League – Division Nine

Blagdon 0   Ratchester . .39

Crowd 4683

In this headline, the number 4683 has been **rounded off to the nearest hundred.**

4683 is between 4600 and 4700.	The halfway mark between 4600 and 4700 is **4650**.	4683 is more than halfway. So it is nearer to **4700** than to 4600.

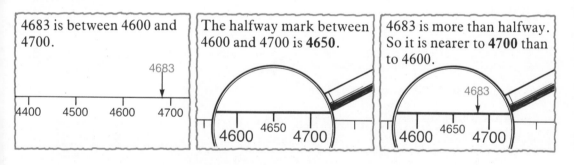

We round off a number when we want to give people a rough idea of the size of the number.

A1 This scale is numbered in hundreds.

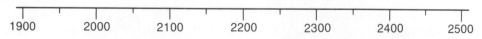

1900   2000   2100   2200   2300   2400   2500

(a) Without marking the scale, point (roughly) to the position of the number 2328 on the scale.
Now round off 2328 to the nearest hundred.

Round off each of these numbers to the nearest hundred.

(b) 2433   (c) 2078   (d) 2107   (e) 2267   (f) 1985

15

The number 2350 is exactly halfway between 2300 and 2400.
When we round off 2350 to the nearest hundred, we usually go 'upwards'.
So 2350 becomes **2400**.

There is a simple rule for rounding off numbers to the nearest hundred.

Pick out the hundreds figure.
If the next figure is 5 or more, round up; otherwise down.

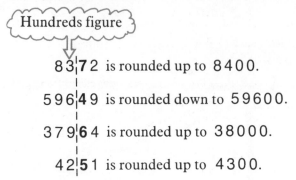

$8\,3\,|\,7\,2$ is rounded up to $8\,4\,0\,0$.

$5\,9\,6\,|\,4\,9$ is rounded down to $5\,9\,6\,0\,0$.

$3\,7\,9\,|\,6\,4$ is rounded up to $3\,8\,0\,0\,0$.

$4\,2\,|\,5\,1$ is rounded up to $4\,3\,0\,0$.

A2   Round these off to the nearest hundred.
(a) 3715   (b) 5876   (c) 4025   (d) 82009   (e) 3971
(f) 2918   (g) 6983   (h) 13625   (i) 18493   (j) 19762

Rounding off to the nearest thousand is similar to rounding off to
the nearest hundred.

Thousands figure

$3\,6\,7\,|\,2\,5\,8$ is rounded down to $3\,6\,7\,0\,0\,0$.

$4\,0\,8\,|\,6\,2\,3$ is rounded up to $4\,0\,9\,0\,0\,0$.

A3   Round these off to the nearest thousand.
(a) 63824   (b) 4159   (c) 23076   (d) 487362   (e) 8530

A4   Round these off to the nearest thousand.   (a) 39756   (b) 649932

A5   Blagdon Town pay a £32785 transfer
fee for the 68 year old veteran striker
Harry Hobble.

This is the newspaper headline.

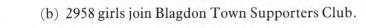

£33,000 WASTED ON CLAPPED-OUT STRIKER !!!

Harry Hobble

Make up headlines for these stories.
Round off the numbers to the nearest thousand.

(a) The manager's wife runs off with £18264 of club money.

(b) 2958 girls join Blagdon Town Supporters Club.

A6 Blagdon Town Football Club is losing money.
This table shows their funds over the past few years.

5 years ago	4 years ago	3 years ago	2 years ago	1 year ago	Now
£462 846	£416 293	£364 593	£311 908	£259 709	£210 037

(a) Copy the table, but round off the amounts to the nearest £1000.

(b) If they carry on losing money like this, after how many more years, roughly, will they run out of money?

A7 Here are the populations of 12 American cities, rounded off to the nearest thousand.

Atlanta	1 390 000	Miami	1 268 000
Baltimore	2 071 000	New Orleans	1 046 000
Chicago	6 979 000	New York	11 572 000
Cleveland	2 064 000	Philadelphia	4 820 000
Detroit	4 200 000	Phoenix	970 000
Houston	1 985 000	Washington	2 861 000

(a) Which cities have a larger population than Baltimore?
(b) What is the population of Chicago, to the nearest million?
(c) What is the population of Cleveland, to the nearest million?
(d) The population of Paris is 2 291 000. Which of the cities in the list above is closest in population to Paris?

B Graphs

B1

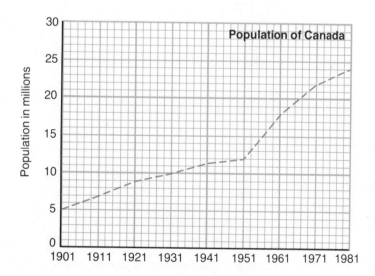

This graph shows how the population of Canada has grown during this century.
From the graph estimate the population, to the nearest million, in

(a) 1911   (b) 1931   (c) 1961   (d) 1971   (e) 1981

Sometimes you have to round off numbers when you draw a graph.

Year	Population (nearest thousand)
1871	27 431 000
1881	31 015 000
1891	34 264 000
1901	38 237 000
1911	42 082 000
1921	44 027 000
1931	46 038 000
1941	No census
1951	50 225 000
1961	52 709 000
1971	55 515 000

The table below shows how the population of the UK has grown since 1871.

This axis is marked in **millions**.

The population in 1871 was 27 million to the nearest million.

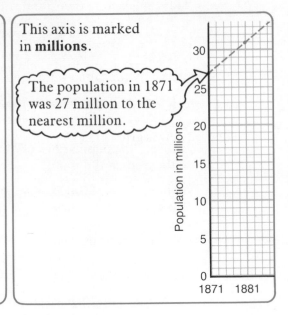

B2 (a) Draw axes as shown above, but go **across** as far as 1981 and **up** to 60 million.
Round off each population figure to the nearest million, and mark it on the graph. (Do not mark a point for 1941.)
Draw a smooth curve through the points.
(b) Use your graph to estimate the population in 1941.
Why was there no census in 1941?

B3 This table shows the population of England and Wales from 1811 to 1971.

Year	Population	Year	Population
1811	10 165 000	1911	36 070 000
1831	13 897 000	1931	39 952 000
1851	17 928 000	1951	43 758 000
1871	22 712 000	1971	48 750 000
1891	29 003 000		

(a) Draw axes like this.
Go **across** to 1971 and **up** to 50 million.

Round off each population figure to the nearest million, and mark it on the graph. Draw a smooth curve through the points.

(b) Estimate the population in
(i) 1841   (ii) 1901   (iii) 1961

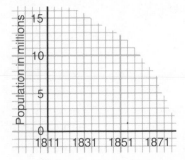

4 Area ②

A Estimating areas

You need tracing paper.

Each square in this grid is 1 cm by 1 cm.
So the area of each square is 1 cm².

It is easy to find the area of this shape,
because it covers an exact number of squares.

Its area is 12 cm².

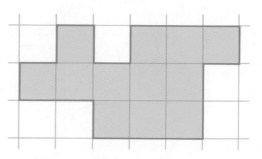

We cannot find the area of this shape
exactly, but we can **estimate** the area.

Put a piece of tracing paper over this
shape. Trace the outline.

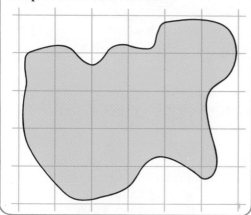

Here is a simple rule for estimating
the area.

If more than half a square
is covered, count it as a
whole square. Mark a dot
on the tracing paper.

If less than half a square
is covered, count it as
nothing. Do not mark a
dot on the tracing paper.

It helps to remember that
this is half a square, ────→

and so is this. ────→

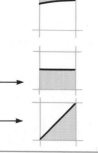

A1 Write down your estimate of the area of the shape above.

A2 Estimate the area
of this shape.
Use tracing paper
and mark dots.

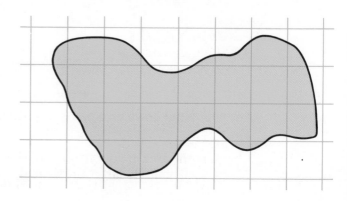

A3 Use the same method to estimate the areas of these animal footprints.

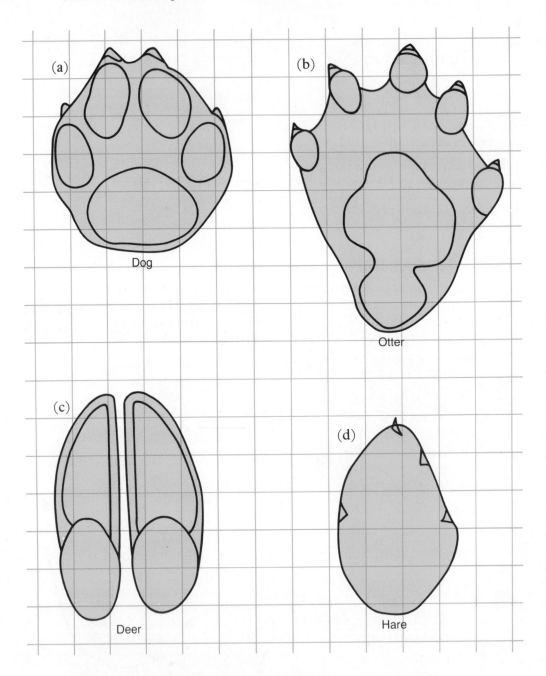

(a) Dog

(b) Otter

(c) Deer

(d) Hare

A4 Put your hand down on a piece of centimetre squared paper. Draw round it, and estimate its area.

Compare the area of your hand with those of other people. Is yours particularly large, or particularly small?

B Different scales

This wild horse's hoof print has been drawn smaller than it really is.

Each grid square stands for, or **represents**, a square 2 cm by 2 cm.

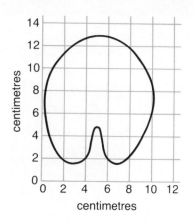

B1 (a) Draw **full size** a grid of squares each 2 cm by 2 cm.
Make your grid 6 squares across and 7 squares up.

Draw the wild horse's hoof print full size on your grid.
Copy the drawing above, and draw the outline square by square, like this.

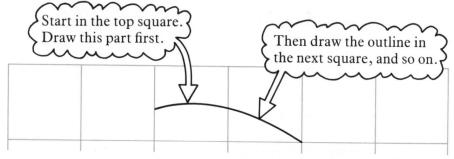

Start in the top square. Draw this part first.

Then draw the outline in the next square, and so on.

(b) What is the area, in cm², of each grid square in your drawing?

(c) Estimate how many grid squares your drawing of the print covers.

(d) Use your answers to (b) and (c) to work out the area of the hoof print, in cm².

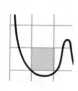

Each square in the small-scale drawing represents 4 cm² in the full-size drawing.

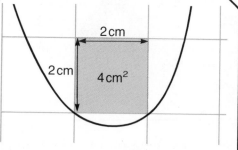

A quicker way to estimate the area of the hoof print is this:
Count the squares in the small-scale drawing. Multiply the number by 4.
What you get is an estimate of the area in cm².

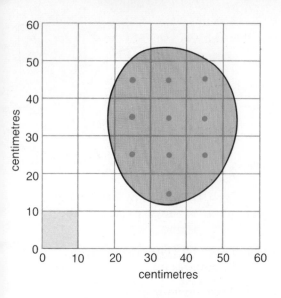

B2 This is a drawing of an elephant's print. There is a dot in each square which is more than half covered by the print.

(a) What area does the grey square represent?

(b) Estimate how many squares the print covers. (Count the dots.)

(c) Estimate the area of the print, using your answers to (a) and (b).

B3 Fossilised dinosaur prints have been found.
A dinosaur very much like the one in the picture made the print below.
An adult human print is shown, to give you an idea of the size.

(a) What area, in cm², does the shaded square represent?

(b) Estimate the number of squares the print covers.

(c) Use your answers to (a) and (b) to estimate the area of the print in cm².

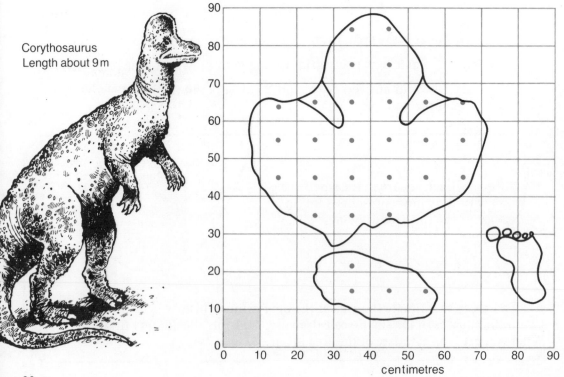

Corythosaurus
Length about 9 m

22

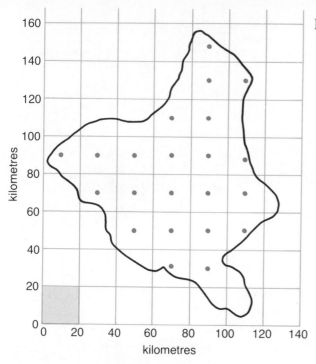

B4 This is a map of the island of Hawaii.

The scale is marked in kilometres, so areas on this map will be in square kilometres (km^2).

(a) What area does the shaded square represent?

(b) Estimate the number of squares covered by the island.

(c) Estimate the area of Hawaii.

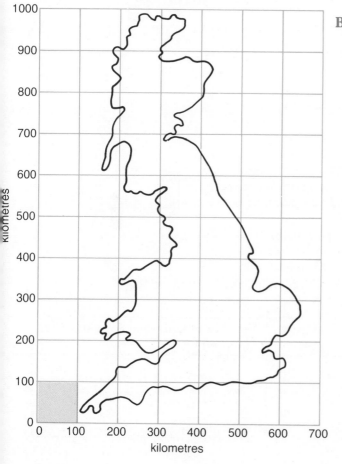

B5 (a) Trace this map of the mainland of Great Britain, and estimate how many squares it covers.

(b) What area does the shaded square represent?

(c) Use your answers to (a) and (b) to estimate the area of the mainland of Great Britain.

(A reference book gives the area as $218\,041\,km^2$. See how close your estimate of the area is to this.)

B6 These pictures of insects are drawn larger than life.
The wings of each insect have been coloured.
The spots show squares which are more than half covered by the wings.

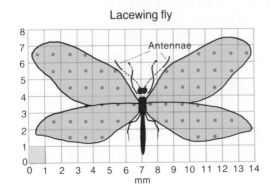

Lacewing fly

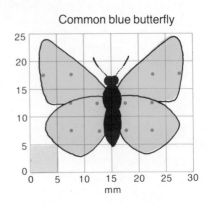

Common blue butterfly

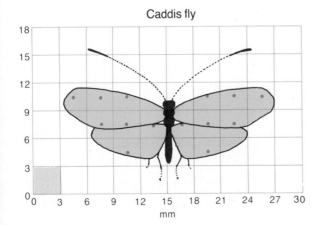

Caddis fly

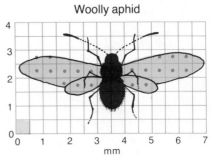

Woolly aphid

(a) Use the scales marked in the pictures
to estimate the wingspan of each insect.
The wingspan is the distance between
the tips of the wings.

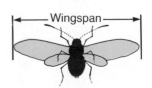

Wingspan

(b) Estimate the length of each insect's body.
(Do not include the antennae.)

(c) Copy and complete this table.
The scales on the drawings are marked in mm, so the
areas will be in mm^2.

Type of insect	Area of grey square	Number of squares covered by wings	Area of wings
Lacewing fly	mm^2		mm^2
Common blue			
Caddis fly			
Woolly aphid			

24

*C Improving the accuracy of area estimates

<table>
<tr>
<td>

Drawing this shape on a 1 cm grid gives a very rough estimate of its area.

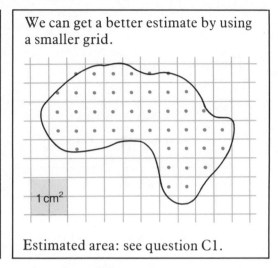

Estimated area: 10 cm²

</td>
<td>

We can get a better estimate by using a smaller grid.

Estimated area: see question C1.

</td>
</tr>
</table>

C1   (a) Count the spotted squares in the second diagram above.

       (b) In the second diagram, 4 spotted squares make 1 cm².
           Use this fact to estimate the area of the shape, in cm².

If the area we want to estimate is large, and the grid squares are small, counting squares is very boring and takes a long time.

It is quicker to mark off rectangles inside the shape, and to calculate the areas of the rectangles.

We still have to count the squares which are left over, but there will not be so many of them.

An example is shown on the right.

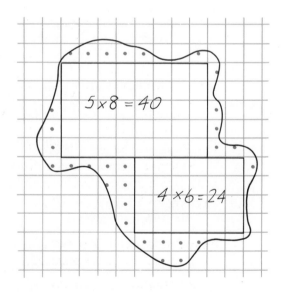

C2   Estimate the area of the shape shown above. (4 squares make 1 cm².)

C3   *You need worksheet B1–2.*

5 Decimals

A Decimal scales: review

A1 This scale is marked in whole numbers and tenths.
Arrow A points to 7·4. What numbers do the other arrows point to?

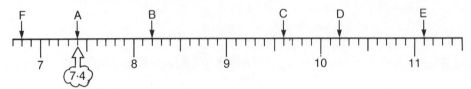

A2 What numbers do these arrows point to?

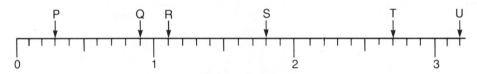

The top scale here goes from 0 to 1 in **tenths**.

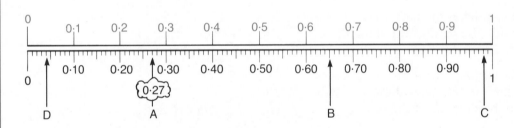

The bottom scale goes from 0 to 1 in **hundredths**.

A3 (a) Arrow A points to 0·27.
What numbers do the other arrows point to?

(b) Notice that 0·20 is equal to 0·2, and that 0·30 equals 0·3.
Notice also that 0·27 is between 0·2 and 0·3, but closer to 0·3.

Copy and complete this sentence, without looking at the scales:

0·83 is between 0·_ and 0·_, but closer to 0·_.

(c) Without looking at the scales, write down the number which is
halfway between 0·1 and 0·2.

A4   Answer these questions **without looking at the scales**.

   (a) Which number is halfway between 0·8 and 0·9?

   (b) Which number is halfway between 0 and 0·1?

   (c) Which number is halfway between 0·9 and 1?

   Now look at the scales and check your answers.

A5   Write these numbers in order of size, smallest first.
   Do not use the scales to help you.

   0·8   0·15   0·3   0·08   0·71   0·9

A6   Without using the scales, write these numbers in order
   of size, smallest first.

   0·33   0·5   0·3   0·40   0·16   0·04

B   Rounding off to the nearest tenth

Look again at the tenths and hundredths scales on the opposite page.
Notice that the nearest 'tenths' mark to 0·27 is 0·3.

If we round off 0·27 **to the nearest tenth,** we get 0·3.

Similarly, if we round off 0·83 to the nearest tenth, we get 0·8,
because 0·8 is the nearest 'tenths' mark to 0·83.

B1   Round these off to the nearest tenth. Do it without looking
   at the scales.

   (a) 0·18   (b) 0·54   (c) 0·62   (d) 0·79   (e) 0·88   (f) 0·22

0·35 is exactly halfway between 0·3 and 0·4.
When we round off 0·35 to the nearest tenth, we usually go 'upwards', to 0·4.

B2   Round these off to the nearest tenth.

   (a) 0·75   (b) 0·15   (c) 0·85   (d) 0·65   (e) 0·45   (f) 0·25

Rounding off to the nearest tenth is also called **rounding off to 1 decimal place** (1 d.p.).

B3   Round these off to 1 d.p.

   (a) 0·29   (b) 0·86   (c) 0·08   (d) 0·34   (e) 0·45   (f) 0·43

*B4   Dawn thinks of a number with two decimal places.
   She rounds it off to 1 decimal place and gives the answer 0·7.

   (a) What is the smallest number Dawn could be thinking of?

   (b) What is the largest number she could be thinking of?

c Numbers with two decimal places

The length of this needle is between 3·7 and 3·8 cm.

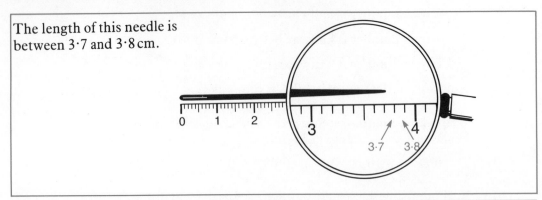

Here is a close-up of the scale between 3·7 and 3·8.

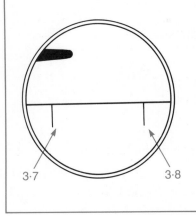

The gap between 3·7 and 3·8 can be divided into 10 equal parts.

The marks are at 3·71, 3·72, 3·73, and so on.

The length of the needle is **3·72 cm.**

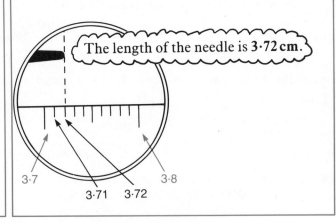

C1 What numbers do each of these arrows point to?

(a)

(b)

(c)

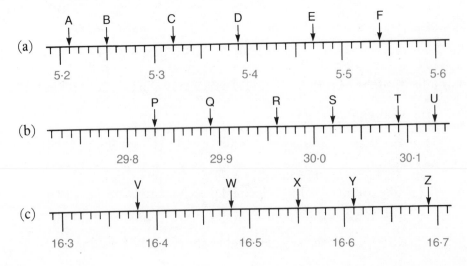

C2 What numbers do these arrows point to?

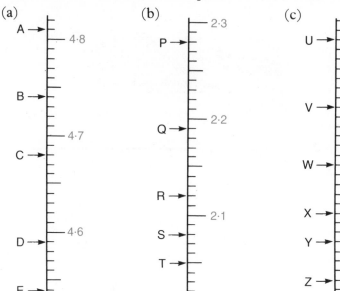

(a)

A →
4·8

B →
4·7

C →

4·6
D →

E →

(b)

2·3
P →

2·2
Q →

R →
2·1

S →

T →

(c)

U →

6·2
V →

W →

6·1
X →

Y →

Z →
6·0

C3 Look at the first of the three scales above.
What number is halfway between 4·6 and 4·7?

C4 What number is halfway between
(a) 3·8 and 3·9   (b) 3·9 and 4·0   (c) 7·9 and 8·0
(d) 6·9 and 7 (Remember that 7 = 7·0.)   (e) 1·9 and 2
(f) 5 and 5·1 (Remember that 5 = 5·0.)   (g) 8 and 8·1

C5 Write down the number which is halfway between
(a) 7·5 and 7·6   (b) 0·8 and 0·9   (c) 0·9 and 1
(d) 14 and 14·1   (e) 26·9 and 27   (f) 1 and 1·1

Rounding off to 1 decimal place

The number 3·76 is between 3·7 and 3·8, but is closer to **3·8**.

When we round off 3·76 to 1 d.p., we get 3·8.

3·73 would be rounded down, to 3·7.

3·75 is rounded up, to 3·8.

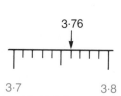

C6 Round off these numbers to 1 d.p.

(a) 8·63   (b) 9·57   (c) 2·33   (d) 1·18   (e) 4·36   (f) 25·89

D Three decimal places

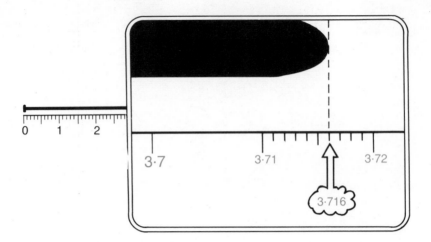

This is a 'super' close-up of a pin being measured.
The length of the pin is between 3·71 and 3·72 cm.

The gap between 3·71 and 3·72 is divided into 10 equal parts, which
go 3·711, 3·712, 3·713, and so on.

The length of the pin is **3·716 cm**.

D1 What numbers do these arrows point to?

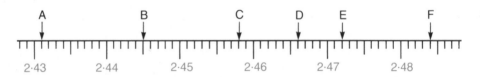

D2 Look at the scale in question D1.
What number is halfway between 2·47 and 2·48?

D3 What number is halfway between

(a) 3·84 and 3·85   (b) 0·78 and 0·79   (c) 0·79 and 0·80

D4 Which is (a) the largest, and (b) the smallest of these numbers?

1·51   1·005   1·055   1·56   1·515

D5 Write these numbers in order, smallest first.

6·32   6·308   6·049   6·269   6·28

Rounding off 'long' decimals

As the number of decimal places increases, so the figures stand for smaller and smaller amounts.

For example, in a reference book it says that **1 gallon** is equal to **4·546 09 litres**.

This is what the figures mean.

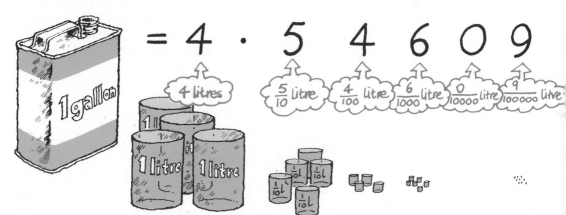

Calculators often give long 'strings' of decimal places.

Usually we do not need to know all the figures, so we round off to 2 d.p. or 3 d.p., etc.

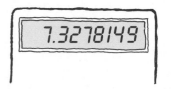

Here is how to round off 7·327 8149 to 2 d.p.

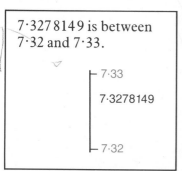

7·3278149 is between 7·32 and 7·33.

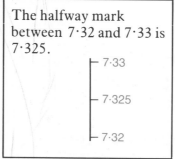

The halfway mark between 7·32 and 7·33 is 7·325.

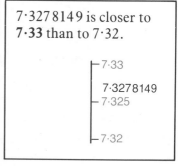

7·3278149 is closer to **7·33** than to 7·32.

When you want to round off to **2 d.p.**, look at the figure in the **3rd** decimal place. If it is 5 or more, round up; otherwise down.

3rd decimal place

7·32|78149 is rounded up to 7·33.

6·18|43708 is rounded down to 6·18.

E1 Round these off to 2 decimal places.

(a) 6·37102   (b) 9·34876   (c) 2·02495   (d) 73·60672

E2 Round off these numbers to 2 decimal places.

(a) 2·0581 (b) 0·873 14 (c) 13·651 03 (d) 2·768 51

See what happens when you round off 3·504 12 to 2 decimal places.

The 3rd decimal place is 4, ... so round **down.**

3·5 0¦4 1 2 ⟶ 3·5 0

This 0 stays, to show that the number was rounded off to 2 decimal places.

E3 Round these off to 2 decimal places.

(a) 7·3023 (b) 12·5008 (c) 11·5068 (d) 8·0026

See what happens when you round off 2·397 to 2 decimal places.

The 3rd decimal place is 7, ... so round **up.**

2·39¦7 ⟶ 2·4 0

Once again, this 0 stays to make 2 decimal places.

E4 Round these off to 2 decimal places.

(a) 4·696 (b) 3·199 (c) 6·098 (d) 2·997

(e) 5·6937 (f) 2·2982 (g) 4·0932 (h) 0·1975

E5 Round these off to 2 decimal places.

(a) 6·598 24 (b) 0·893 71 (c) 4·399 86 (d) 5·097 51

(e) 8·390 95 (f) 5·996 24 (g) 2·897 15 (h) 0·998 63

E6 Round these off to 1 decimal place.

(a) 8·634 78 (b) 2·495 73 (c) 0·876 11 (d) 2·981 36

(e) 9·826 17 (f) 8·970 23 (g) 8·613 04 (h) 9·960 27

E7 Round these off to 3 decimal places.

(a) 5·326 81 (b) 4·070 95 (c) 2·098 73 (d) 4·189 58

4.3972087

E8 Round off the number in this calculator display to

(a) 1 d.p. (b) 2 d.p. (c) 3 d.p.

(d) 4 d.p. (e) 5 d.p. (f) 6 d.p.

F Estimating

F1 Copy this scale exactly. (Either trace it, or put the edge of a piece of paper against it.)

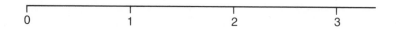

(a) Mark an arrow on your scale where you think 1·5 would be. Do not measure; estimate the position of 1·5. Label your arrow '1·5'.

(b) Do the same for 0·4, 1·9, 2·8, 3·3.

Check your answers from the scale at the bottom of the next page.

These pictures show where the different 'tenths' marks are between 0 and 1.

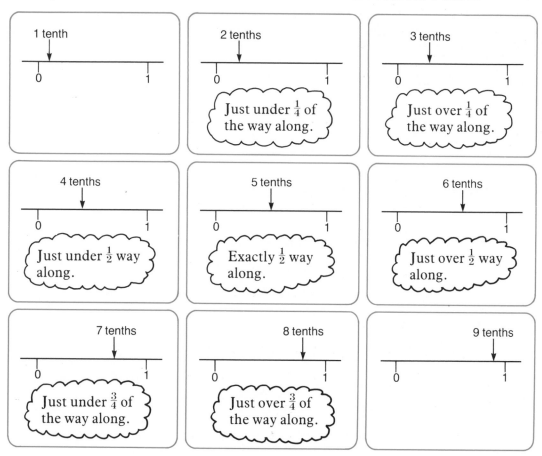

Look through these diagrams carefully, before you turn over.

Do these questions without looking at the diagrams on the previous page.

F2 Estimate, to 1 decimal place, the numbers which these arrows point to.

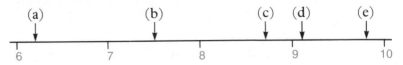

F3 Estimate, to 1 d.p., the numbers which these arrows point to.

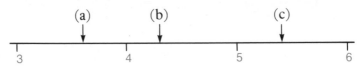

F4 This arrow points to a number between 6·3 and 6·4.

Estimate the number to 2 decimal places.

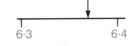

F5 Estimate, to 2 d.p., the numbers marked by arrows.

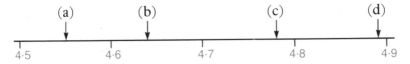

F6 Estimate, to 2 d.p., the numbers marked by arrows.

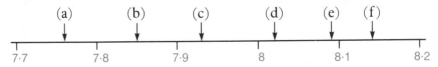

Answer to question F1

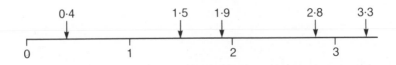

1 Area (1)

1.1 Calculate the area of each of these floor plans.

(a)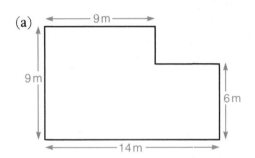

(b)

1.2 Work these out, without using a calculator.

    (a) 50×70 (b) 3×80 (c) 40×50 (d) 60×30 (e) 30×30

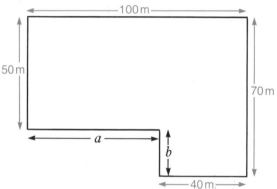

1.3 Without using a calculator, find

    (a) the length marked a

    (b) the length marked b

    (c) the area of the shape

1.4 Without using a calculator, work out the area of

    (a) a rectangle 40 cm by 30 cm

    (b) a square whose sides are each 50 cm long

    (c) a square whose sides are each 80 cm long

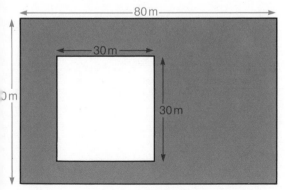

1.5 Calculate the shaded area in this diagram, without using a calculator.

2 Patterns (1)

2.1 Copy each of these drawings and complete it so that the dotted line is a line of reflection symmetry.

(a)  (b) (c)

2.2 Copy this drawing and complete it so that both dotted lines are lines of reflection symmetry.

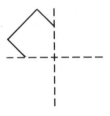

2.3 If you reflect this design in the dotted line,

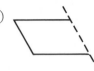

which of these will you see?

A  B 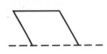 C  D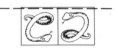

2.4 Which of these designs have a 2-fold rotation centre?

A 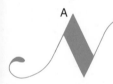 B 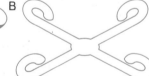 C 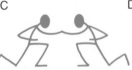 D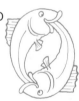

2.5 Copy each of these drawings and complete it so that C is a 2-fold rotation centre.

(a)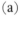

(b)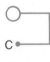

3 Rounding

3.1 Round off these numbers to the nearest hundred.
   (a) 25 431   (b) 48 763   (c) 972 685   (d) 40 709
   (e) 30 085   (f) 29 965   (g) 1578   (h) 2 693 658

3.2 Round off these numbers to the nearest thousand.
   (a) 28 672   (b) 19 543   (c) 18 267   (d) 205 491
   (e) 60 073   (f) 5 284 819 (g) 8 372 655 (h) 69 928

4 Area (2)

4.1 This is a map of a lake.

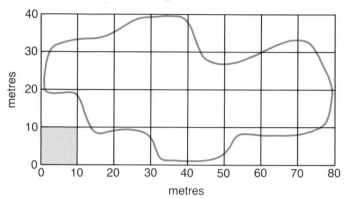

(a) What area does the shaded square represent?

(b) Count the squares covered by the lake. (Tracing paper may help.)

(c) Estimate the area of the lake.

4.2 This is a map of an island. There is a dot in each square which is more than half covered by the island.

(a) What area does the shaded square represent?

(b) Estimate the area of the island.

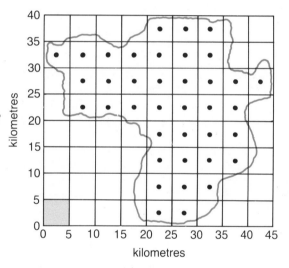

4.3 Estimate the area of each of these islands.

(a)

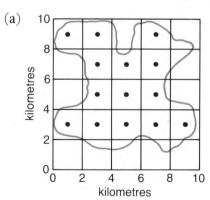

(b)

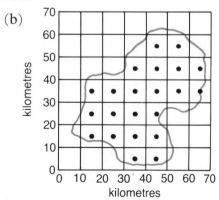

5 Decimals

5.1 Write down the numbers which these arrows point to.

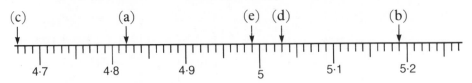

5.2 Which number is halfway between
  (a) 6·7 and 6·8   (b) 4 and 4·1   (c) 3·63 and 3·64

5.3 Round off each of these numbers to 1 decimal place.
  (a) 8·472   (b) 3·086   (c) 2·519   (d) 4·962   (e) 0·509

5.4 Round off each of these numbers to 2 decimal places.
  (a) 6·2738   (b) 4·1986   (c) 0·0342   (d) 5·5031   (e) 1·14778

M Miscellaneous

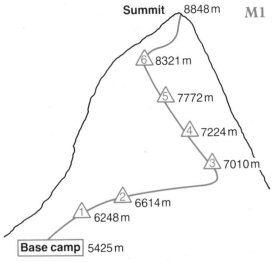

M1 This diagram shows the camps set up during the ascent of the south-west face of Everest in 1975.

(a) Base camp was set up at a height of 5425 metres. What is the difference in height between base camp and the summit?

(b) What is the height still to be climbed from camp 6?

(c) What is the difference in height between camps 2 and 3?

(d) Which two camps have the smallest difference in height between them?

M2

(a) Round off the heights of these mountains to the nearest 100 m.

Mont Blanc	4807 m
Ben Nevis	1343 m
Scafell Pike	978 m
The Cheviot	816 m
Everest	8848 m

(b) If 1 mm stands for 100 m, then this line shows the height of Mont Blanc.

Draw this line. Draw other lines next to it for the other mountains.

48 mm

Label the lines.

Mont Blanc

M3 A sheet of card is 20 cm by 40 cm.

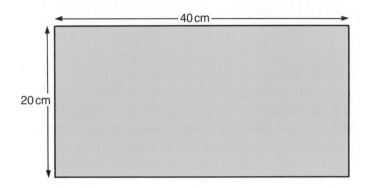

Ranjit has to cut out tickets from the sheet of card.
Each ticket has to be 3 cm by 4 cm.

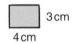 3 cm

4 cm

(a) Here is one way to cut them out.

How many tickets will there be
if they are cut out in this way?
(Some of the card will be wasted.)

(b) Here is another way to cut them out.

How many tickets will there be if
they are cut out in this way?

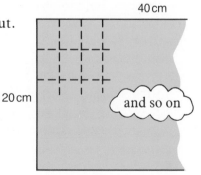

(c) Which of the two ways of cutting
will give Ranjit more tickets and
less waste?

M4 As question M3, but this time the sheet of card is 50 cm by 100 cm,
and the tickets are 3 cm by 7 cm.

6 Multiplication

A Multiplying decimals

If material costs £1·50 a metre and you want 3 metres, then you work out the total cost by **multiplying** £1·50 by 3.

$$£1·50 × 3 = £4·50$$

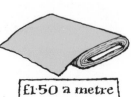

£1·50 a metre

And if you want 4 metres, you have to multiply £1·50 by 4.

$$£1·50 × 4 = £6·00$$

Suppose you want 3·6 metres.

3·6 metres is somewhere between 3 metres and 4 metres.
So the cost of 3·6 metres will be somewhere between £4·50 and £6·00.

To work out the cost of 3·6 metres, you multiply £1·50 by 3·6.

3·6 m

£1·50 a metre

$$£1·50 × 3·6 = £5·40$$

A1 (a) Find the cost of 5 metres of electric cable at £1·80 a metre.

(b) Find the cost of 6 metres of the same cable.

(c) Find the cost of 5·3 metres of the same cable.
Check that the answer is somewhere between the answers to parts (a) and (b).

A2 Pat wants to buy 7·8 metres of curtain material which costs £4 a metre. She knows, without using her calculator, that the total cost must be less than £32.

(a) How does she know this?

(b) Calculate the cost of 7·8 metres of the material.

A3 (a) Calculate the cost of 4·6 metres of dress material at £5·95 a metre.

(b) How can you tell before doing the calculation that the cost must be less than £30?

Many shops use **ready reckoners**.

They are tables giving the answers to calculations which the shop assistants often have to do.

Here is part of a ready reckoner which gives the costs of various lengths of material at different prices per metre.

metres	Price per metre				
	£2·40	£2·50	£2·60	£2·70	£2·80
3·00	£7·20	£7·50	£7·80	£8·10	£8·40
3·10	£7·44	£7·75	£8·06	£8·37	£8·68
3·20	£7·68	£8·00	£8·32	£8·64	£8·96
3·30	£7·92	£8·25	£8·58	£8·91	£9·24
3·40	£8·16	£8·50	£8·84	£9·18	£9·52
3·50	£8·40	£8·75	£9·10	£9·45	£9·80
3·60	£8·64	£9·00	£9·36	£9·72	

A4 Use the ready reckoner to find the cost of each of these.

(a) 3·20 metres at £2·40 per metre

(b) 3·50 metres at £2·70 per metre

(c) 3 metres at £2·80 per metre

A5 Canvas costs £2·60 a metre.

(a) How can you tell from the ready reckoner that 3·45 metres of canvas will cost somewhere between £8·84 and £9·10?

(b) Use a calculator to work out the cost of 3·45 metres of canvas.

A6 The amount in the bottom right-hand corner of the picture above is missing. Use a calculator to work out the missing amount.

A7 Look at the column for '£2·40 per metre'.
Suppose this column is continued downwards to show the cost of 3·70 m, 3·80 m, and so on.

Work out the costs of 3·70 m, 3·80 m, and so on up to 4 m.

A8 (a) Use the ready reckoner to help you complete this sentence.

The cost of 3·05 m at £2·80 per metre is somewhere between £ . . . and £ . . .

(b) Use a calculator to work out the cost of 3·05 m at £2·80 per metre.

A9 How can you use the ready reckoner to find the cost of 6·40 m of material at £2·40 per metre?

There are different ways of using the reckoner to find the cost of 6·40 m. Try to think of **two** different ways.
Make sure they both give the same answer.

Check that the answer is correct by multiplying on a calculator.

Rounding off to the nearest penny

The cheese on this weighing machine costs £1·84 per kilogram.

The piece of cheese weighs 1·7 kg.

To find what it costs we work out

£1·84 × 1·7.

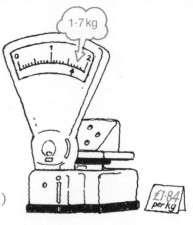

The answer we get on a calculator is £3·128. (Check this.)
We round off this amount to the nearest penny.

The 3rd decimal place is 5 or more, . . . so we round up.

£3·12|8 ⟶ £3·13   to the nearest penny

A10   Round off these amounts to the nearest penny.

(a) £6·532   (b) £8·408   (c) £6·379 64   (d) £4·073 95

(e) £7·697   (f) £3·5882   (g) £7·8509   (h) £1·9962

A11   Work out the total cost of each of these pieces of meat.
Round off each one to the nearest penny.

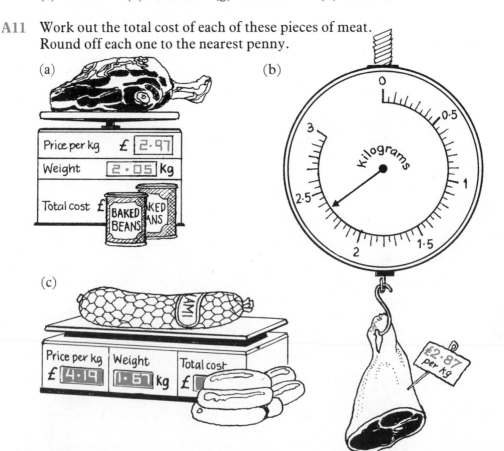

(a)

Price per kg	£	2·97
Weight	2·05	kg
Total cost	£	

(b)

(c)

| Price per kg | Weight | Total cost |
| £ 4·19 | 1·67 kg | £ |

£2·87 per kg

42

B Multiplying by a number less than 1

The cheese on this weighing machine costs £1·75 per kilogram.

The cheese weighs 0·6 kg, and the machine shows that 0·6 kg costs £1·05.

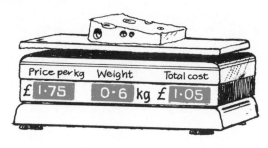

Check with a calculator that

£1·75 × 0·6 = £1·05.

When you multiply a number by 0·6, the answer is smaller than the number you started with.

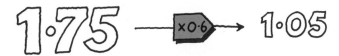

0·6 kilogram is less than 1 kilogram, so the cost of 0·6 kilogram must be less than the cost of 1 kilogram.

B1 Calculate the cost of each of these to the nearest penny. Before you do each one, ask yourself whether the answer will be **more** than the cost of 1 kilogram, or **less** than the cost of 1 kilogram.

(a) 0·8 kg of meat at £1·90 per kg

(b) 1·2 kg of bananas at £1·15 per kg

(c) 0·65 kg of cod at £2·05 per kg

B2 1 metre of silk material costs £4·80.
So 0·5 metre costs £4·80 × 0·5 = £2·40.

This scale shows the cost of 1 metre and the cost of 0·5 m.

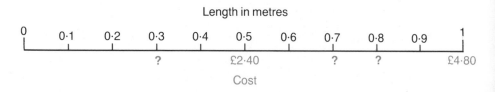

(a) Calculate the cost of 0·3 m of the material.

(b) Calculate the cost of 0·7 m.

(c) Calculate the cost of 0·8 m.

(d) Without using a calculator, write down the cost of 0·1 m.

43

When you multiply something by a number less than 1, you make it smaller.

For example, 84×0.3 must be less than 84,

$\qquad 0.9 \times 32$ (or 32×0.9) must be less than 32.

When you multiply something by a number greater than 1, you make it bigger.

B3 The missing word in each of these sentences is either 'greater' or 'less'. Without using a calculator, say what each missing word should be.

(a) 2.4×1.06 is . . . . . than 2.4.

(b) 53.6×0.89 is . . . . . than 53.6.

(c) 0.96×7.05 is . . . . . than 7.05.

(d) 0.96×7.05 is . . . . . than 0.96.

(e) 0.68×0.51 is . . . . . than 0.51.

(f) 0.68×0.51 is . . . . . than 0.68.

This calculation must be wrong, because the answer must be bigger than 58. $58 \times 1.37 = 52.46$ ✗	This calculation must be wrong, because the answer must be smaller than 62. $0.43 \times 62 = 78.16$ ✗

B4 Put the calculator away for this question.
Which of these calculations must be wrong?

(a) $67 \times 1.35 = 58.6$ (b) $73.2 \times 0.8 = 116.4$ (c) $38.5 \times 0.24 = 9.24$
(d) $147 \times 0.3 = 152.6$ (e) $4.8 \times 0.72 = 3.456$ (f) $0.97 \times 0.7 = 0.679$

B5 Calculate the number that comes out at the end of this machine chain.

In 400 —[$\times 0.6$]—[$\times 0.6$]—[$\times 0.6$]—[$\times 0.6$]→ Out

B6 Enter 100 into your calculator.
Multiply by 0.9, press '=' and count 'one' to yourself.
Multiply by 0.9 again, press '=' and count 'two'.

Continue like this. How many times do you have to multiply by 0.9 to get a number which is less than 10?

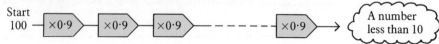

Start 100 —[$\times 0.9$]—[$\times 0.9$]—[$\times 0.9$]— – – – – –[$\times 0.9$]→ (A number less than 10)

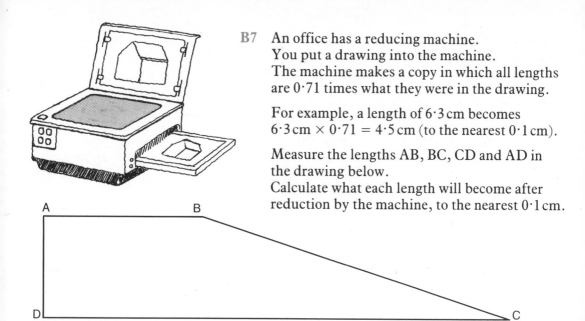

B7 An office has a reducing machine.
You put a drawing into the machine.
The machine makes a copy in which all lengths
are 0·71 times what they were in the drawing.

For example, a length of 6·3 cm becomes
6·3 cm × 0·71 = 4·5 cm (to the nearest 0·1 cm).

Measure the lengths AB, BC, CD and AD in
the drawing below.
Calculate what each length will become after
reduction by the machine, to the nearest 0·1 cm.

HUNDRED UP

This is a game for 2 players, with one calculator between them.

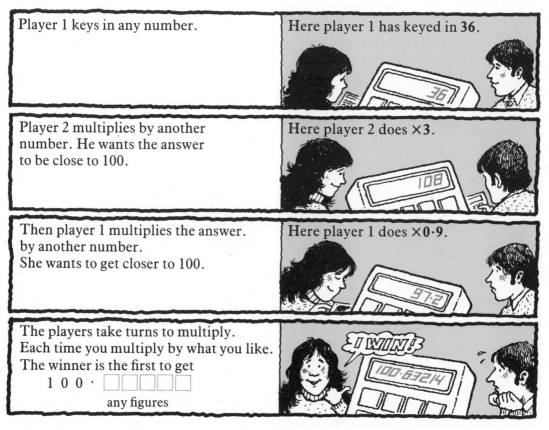

Player 1 keys in any number.	Here player 1 has keyed in **36**.
Player 2 multiplies by another number. He wants the answer to be close to 100.	Here player 2 does ×**3**.
Then player 1 multiplies the answer. by another number. She wants to get closer to 100.	Here player 1 does ×**0·9**.
The players take turns to multiply. Each time you multiply by what you like. The winner is the first to get 100 · ☐☐☐☐☐ any figures	

c Rough answers

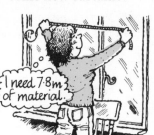

Kathy wanted to make some new curtains.

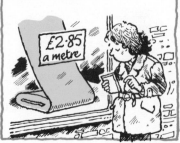

She worked out what it would cost . . .

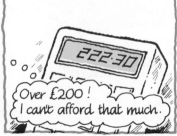

and decided she couldn't afford it.

If Kathy had thought about it, she would have known she had made a mistake somewhere.

£2·85 a metre is roughly £3 a metre.
7·8 metres is roughly 8 metres.
So the total cost is roughly £3 × 8 = £24.

When you use a calculator, **use your brain as well!**
If you have a rough idea of the answer, you won't write down a silly answer.

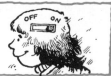

C1   Do not use a calculator!
Choose which of the four numbers is closest to the answer to each calculation.

(a) $4·95 \times 3·16$ 7   12   15   25

(b) $8·14 \times 0·42$ 3   12   30   300

(c) $7·13 \times 2·88$ 14   21   63   200

(d) $0·86 \times 5·12$ 4   6   8   10

(e) The cost of 6·2 metres of material at £3·45 per metre
    £6   £9   £18   £30

(f) The cost of 13·4 metres of plastic tubing at £0·53 per metre
    £5   £7   £12   £20

C2   Use a calculator to check your answers to question C1.

C3   Without using a calculator, write down which of these calculations are obviously wrong.

(a) $6·9 \times 3·21 = 14·609$ (b) $8·04 \times 4·8 = 38·592$
(c) $10·2 \times 15·8 = 131·16$ (d) $0·88 \times 7·34 = 18·642$
(e) $0·47 \times 6·4 = 3·008$ (f) $5·87 \times 5·26 = 308·762$

You can get a rough answer to $4 \cdot 8 \times 6 \cdot 3$ like this.

4·8 is between 4 and 5, but closer to **5**.

6·3 is between 6 and 7, but closer to **6**.

So $4 \cdot 8 \times 6 \cdot 3$ is **roughly** 5×6, or **30**.

C4 Do not use a calculator.
Write down a rough answer for each of these.

(a) $3 \cdot 1 \times 8 \cdot 7$ (b) $6 \cdot 2 \times 1 \cdot 9$ (c) $3 \cdot 1 \times 4 \cdot 3$

(d) $7 \cdot 71 \times 4 \cdot 23$ (e) $3 \cdot 24 \times 5 \cdot 87$ (f) $9 \cdot 87 \times 3 \cdot 78$

(g) $1 \cdot 07 \times 4 \cdot 92$ (h) $7 \cdot 04 \times 4 \cdot 13$ (i) $0 \cdot 96 \times 3 \cdot 34$

C5 Use a calculator to find the exact answer to each part of question C4.

C6 You can get a rough answer to $28 \cdot 3 \times 5 \cdot 93$ like this.
$28 \cdot 3$ is between 20 and 30, but closer to **30**.
$5 \cdot 93$ is between 5 and 6, but closer to **6**.
So $28 \cdot 3 \times 5 \cdot 93$ is roughly $30 \times 6 = \mathbf{180}$.

Write down a rough answer for each of these.

(a) $42 \cdot 3 \times 3 \cdot 85$ (b) $87 \cdot 6 \times 2 \cdot 05$ (c) $31 \cdot 5 \times 6 \cdot 78$

(d) $4 \cdot 88 \times 53 \cdot 1$ (e) $2 \cdot 33 \times 34 \cdot 2$ (f) $7 \cdot 16 \times 58 \cdot 6$

(g) $68 \cdot 9 \times 3 \cdot 77$ (h) $4 \cdot 09 \times 43 \cdot 2$ (i) $62 \cdot 4 \times 2 \cdot 89$

C7 Use a calculator to find the exact answer to each part of question C6.

D Calculator problems

Before you write down an answer, think about it.
Make sure it is a sensible answer to the problem.

D1 1 metre of rubber tubing costs £0·40 and weighs 0·3 kg.

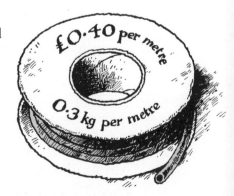

(a) How much does 2·5 metres cost?

(b) How much does 2·5 metres weigh?

(c) How much does 0·8 m cost?

(d) How much does 0·8 m weigh?

47

D2 This is part of a ready reckoner
for finding the cost of silver wire.

1 metre of wire costs £5·60.

(a) One of the costs in the table is wrong.
How can you tell straight away
which one is wrong, without using
a calculator?

(b) Work out what that cost should be.

Length in m.	Cost
0.4	£2.24
0.8	£5.88
1.2	£6.72
1.6	£8.96

Paying for electricity

When an electric fire is left on for a time, it uses up a number of
units of electricity.

To find the number of units, you multiply the **power** of the fire (in
kilowatts) by the number of hours it is used.

The power is printed on a label on the fire.

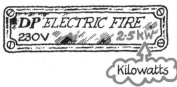

Number of units = power in kilowatts × time in hours

D3 A 2·5 kW electric fire is on for 6 hours.
How many units of electricity does it use up?

This table gives the powers (in kilowatts) of some other electrical appliances.

Fan heater	2 kW	Fridge	0·15 kW
Tumble dryer	2·7 kW	100-watt light bulb	0·1 kW
Iron	1·01 kW	60-watt light bulb	0·06 kW

D4 Calculate the number of units used up when
(a) the fan heater is left on for 8 hours
(b) the tumble dryer is left on for $3\frac{1}{2}$ hours
(c) the fridge is left on for 72 hours

D5 If electricity cost 5p per unit, calculate the cost of
the electricity used in each part of question D4. (Round off
to the nearest penny, if necessary.)

D6 If electricity costs 5p per unit, calculate the cost of
the electricity used up when
(a) the fan heater is left on for 5 hours
(b) the fridge is left on for 120 hours
(c) the tumble dryer is left on for $\frac{3}{4}$ hour
(d) a 100-watt bulb is left on for 12 hours

E Calculating areas

We calculate the area of a rectangle by multiplying the length by the width.

If the length and width are decimals, then it is useful to have a rough idea of the area before doing the calculation.

This rectangle is 4·3 cm by 1·8 cm.

If we round off to the nearest cm, then the rectangle is roughly 4 cm by 2 cm.

So we would expect its area to be about 8 cm².

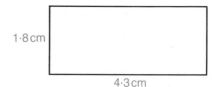

E1 Calculate the area of the rectangle above.

E2 Write down a rough value for the area of each of these rectangles. Then calculate the area and round it off to the nearest 0·1 cm².

(a) 6·2 cm by 4·9 cm   (b) 3·8 cm by 5·7 cm

(c) 9·9 cm by 14·1 cm   (d) 7·3 cm by 7·7 cm

E3 Aisha lives in a flat. A plan of the flat is drawn below.
The scale of the plan is **1 cm to 1 metre**.

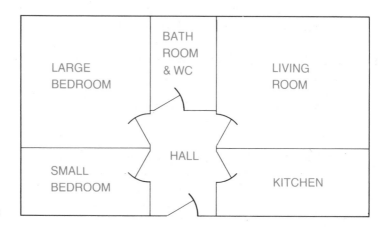

Scale
1 cm to 1 m

(a) Measure the length and width of each room, and calculate the area of each room, to the nearest 0·1 m².

(b) Aisha has 2 litres of white emulsion paint. She wants to paint the ceilings of some of the rooms. (The ceilings have the same areas as the floors.) 1 litre of paint will cover about 12 m².

What combinations of rooms could Aisha paint without having to buy more paint? (For example, could she paint the large bedroom and the living room?)

7 Investigations

A Number chains

This is a 'number chain'.

You get the number in each
square box by adding up the
two numbers on either side
of it.

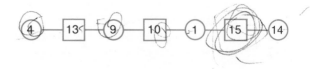

For example, $13 = 4 + 9$.

A1 Leave the numbers in the square boxes as they are.

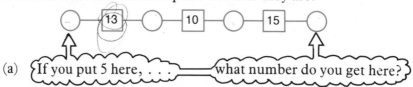

(a) 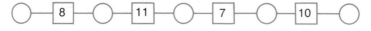 If you put 5 here, . . . what number do you get here?

(b) Try some different starting numbers, and find the finishing
number each time. Make a table like this.

Starting number	Finishing number

Is there any rule connecting the starting and finishing numbers?
If so, write down what the rule is.

(c) Can you make the starting number equal to the finishing number?
What must the starting number be?

A2 Now you have a longer chain.

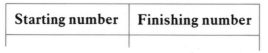

Experiment with this chain.

Can you find a number to put at the start so as to get the
same number at the end? Explain.

A3 Draw a chain with six round boxes and five square ones.
Write a number in each square box.

See if you can find a starting number which is equal to the
number at the end of the chain.

B Closed chains

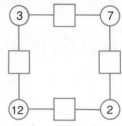

B1 This is a closed chain with four boxes of each kind.

What numbers go in the square boxes?

B2 (a) Draw some more closed chains with four boxes of each kind. Put numbers into each one.

(b) Take any of the chains you have made.
Add up the numbers in the square boxes.
Add up the numbers in the round boxes.

What do you notice? Is it always true?
Can you explain why it is always true?

B3 Can you find the missing numbers here? Is there more than one possible set of missing numbers?

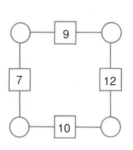

B4 Can you find the missing numbers here?

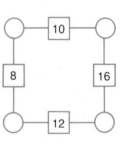

B5 (a) Make some chains with three boxes of each kind, and put numbers into each one.

(b) Choose one of your chains.
Add up the numbers in round boxes, and the numbers in square boxes.
Compare the answers. What do you notice?
Is it true for the other chains you made?

(c) Find the missing numbers in this chain. Describe how you do it, step by step.

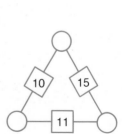

51

8 Division

A The division sign: a reminder

The sign ÷ means **divided by**.

$15 \div 3$ and $3 \div 15$ mean two completely different things.

$15 \div 3$ means '15 divided by 3', and the answer is 5.

$3 \div 15$ means '3 divided by 15', and the answer is **not** 5.

A1 Without using a calculator, say which of these give the answer 4.
Write 'yes' or 'no' for each one.

(a) $2 \div 8$ (b) $16 \div 4$ (c) $20 \div 5$ (d) $5 \div 20$

(e) $24 \div 6$ (f) $10 \div 40$ (g) $8 \div 32$ (h) $1 \div 4$

A2 Without using a calculator, say whether these are right or wrong.

(a) $3 \div 6 = 2$ (b) $40 \div 5 = 8$ (c) $25 \div 5 = 5$ (d) $8 \div 16 = 2$
(e) $7 \div 7 = 1$ (f) $3 \div 18 = 6$ (g) $30 \div 6 = 5$ (h) $1 \div 3 = 3$

B Using a calculator

This pile of books is 63 cm high.

There are 18 books in the pile, and each book has the same thickness.

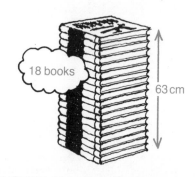
18 books
63 cm

If you want to calculate the thickness of each book, you have to **divide 63 cm by 18**.

On a calculator, you do

$63 \div 18$

The number you are **dividing by** comes second, after the ÷ sign.

The answer to $63 \div 18$ is 3·5. So each book is **3·5 cm thick**.

Checking You can check the answer by multiplying 3·5 cm by 18.
You should get the total height 63 cm.

$$3 \cdot 5 \times 18 = 63 \ \checkmark$$

Check the answers to the questions below by multiplying.

B1 15 people join together to enter a football pool. They agree to share out any winnings equally between them.
They win a total of £7200.
Calculate the amount each person gets.

B2 Another group wins a total of £6510. There are 14 people in this group, and they share winnings equally.
How much does each person get?

B3 24 identical drainpipes are laid end to end to make a total length of 33·6 metres. How long is each drainpipe?

B4 Shaheena worked for 41 hours in a week and was paid £100.
How much was she paid for each hour, to the nearest penny?

C Dividing a number by a larger number

In all the problems so far, you have divided by the smaller number.
This is not always the right thing to do.

There are 8 identical bricks on this weighing machine.

Their total weight is 6 kilograms.

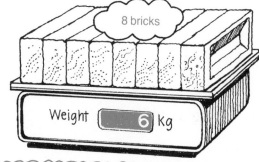

If you want to calculate the weight of each brick, you have to **divide 6 kg by 8**.

On a calculator, you do

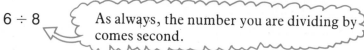

$$6 \div 8$$ As always, the number you are dividing by comes second.

The answer to $6 \div 8$ is 0·75. So each brick weighs **0·75 kg**.

This is a sensible answer, because if 8 bricks weigh 6 kg altogether, each brick must weigh less than 1 kg.

Checking You can check the answer by multiplying. $0·75 \times 8 = 6$ ✓

C1 16 identical rods have a total length of 10 metres. Calculate the length of each rod. Check by multiplying.

C2 8 kg of fruit is to be shared out equally between 25 people.
How much will each person get? Check by multiplying.

C3 A choir of 15 children enter a singing contest and win a prize of £12, which they agree to share equally.

(a) Which of these calculations gives the amount each child gets, $15 \div 12$ or $12 \div 15$?

(b) Calculate the amount each child gets. Check your answer by multiplying.

C4 250 identical ball-bearings have a total weight of 1850 grams. Which of these calculations gives the weight of one ball-bearing, $250 \div 1850$ or $1850 \div 250$?

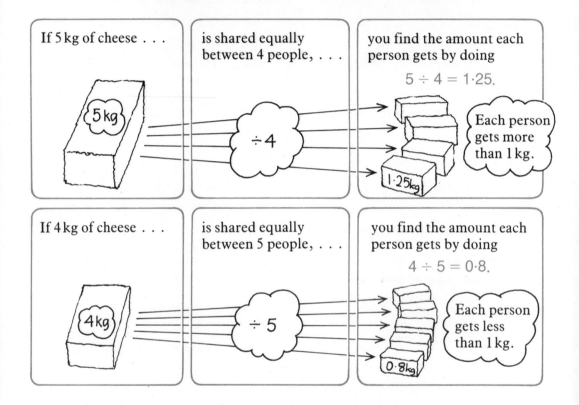

If you divide a number by a smaller number, the answer is greater than 1.

If you divide a number by a larger number, the answer is less than 1.

In questions C5 to C11, be careful to divide the numbers the right way round. Think whether the answer should be greater or less than 1.

C5 4 people share £3 equally between them.
(a) Do they get more, or less, than £1 each?
(b) How much does each person get?

C6 (a) A metal strip 10 m long is cut into 8 equal pieces.
How long is each piece?
(b) Another strip 8 m long is cut into 10 equal pieces.
How long is each piece?

C7 16 identical cannon balls weigh 14 kg altogether.
How much does 1 ball weigh?

C8 A pile of books is 17 cm high.
There are 25 books in the pile and they are all the same thickness.
How thick is each book?

C9 64 fiftypence coins weigh 864 grams. How much does
one coin weigh?

C10 250 sheets of paper have a total thickness of 3·6 cm.
How thick is 1 sheet?

C11 A water pipe weighs 46 kg and is 40 m long.
How much does 1 metre of the pipe weigh?

D Unit costs

This 3 kg bag of potatoes costs 96p.

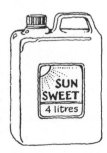

If you pay 96p for 3 kg, then you can
find the cost of each kilogram by dividing
96p by 3.

96p ÷ 3 = 32p.

The cost of 1 kilogram is called the **cost per kilogram** of the
potatoes.

D1 A 2 kg bag of onions costs 74p.
Calculate the cost per kilogram of the onions.

D2 In a shop you pay £2·85 for a bag containing 3 kg of
barbecue fuel.

Calculate the cost per kilogram of the fuel.

D3 A supermarket sells cartons of
orange drink, which contain 4 litres.

They cost £1·45 each.

How much does a customer pay for
each litre of orange drink in the carton,
to the nearest penny?

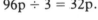

55

Which of these bags is better value?

To answer this question you need to find out what you are paying for 1 kg of seed in each bag.

In other words, you calculate the cost per kilogram of the grass seed in each bag.

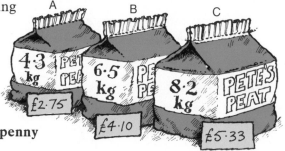

D4 (a) In the small bag,
3 kg of seed costs £2·55.
What does 1 kg cost?

(b) Find the cost per kilogram of the large bag.

(c) Which bag is better value?

You find the cost per kilogram by dividing the cost by the weight in kg.

To find the cost per kilogram of bag A you need to do £2·75 ÷ 4·3.

When you do this on a calculator, you get £0·6395348 . . .

When you round this off to the **nearest penny** you get **£0·64**.

D5 (a) Calculate the cost per kilogram of bag B, to the nearest penny.

(b) Do the same for bag C.

(c) Which of the bags A, B and C is the best value?

D6 The pictures below show pairs of items.
Calculate the cost per kilogram of each item.
Say which of the items in each pair is better value.

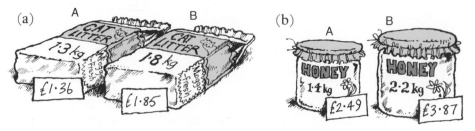

D7 A supermarket sells lemonade in two sizes of bottle.
The smaller bottle holds 1·5 litres and costs 57p.
The larger bottle holds 2·5 litres and costs £1.

Calculate the cost per litre of the lemonade in each bottle.

Different kinds of things are measured in different **units**, such as kilograms, litres, metres, etc.

The cost of 1 unit (it may be 1 kg, or 1 litre, or 1 metre, etc.) is called the **unit cost**.

For example, if a 2-litre bottle of orange drink costs 46p, the unit cost of the drink is **23p per litre**.

Unit cost = cost ÷ weight, or volume, or length, etc.

D8 Calculate the unit cost of each item in the pairs below.
Compare the 'value for money' of the items in each pair.

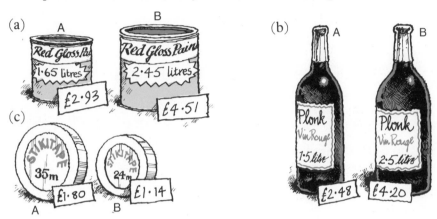

D9 A shop sells cheese in large blocks weighing 2 kg and costing £4·50.

Another shop sells 1 kg pieces of cheese at £2·50.

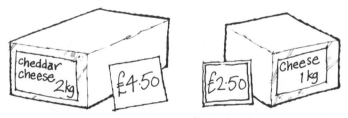

The unit cost of the first cheese is £2·25 per kg.
The unit cost of the second cheese is £2·50 per kg.

It is fair to compare these unit costs only if the cheese is of the same quality in both shops.

Suppose the cheese is of the same quality in both shops. Can you think of any reasons why someone might prefer to buy a 1 kg piece rather than a 2 kg piece, even though the larger piece is 'better value for money'?

E Problems needing multiplication or division

E1 Do not use a calculator for this question.

A pile of 25 identical textbooks is 72 cm high, and each textbook weighs 0·28 kg.

Which of the calculations below would you do to find

(a) the thickness of one textbook

(b) the total weight of the pile

72 ÷ 0·28	25 × 0·28	25 ÷ 72	25 ÷ 0·28
72 ÷ 25	0·28 ÷ 25	0·28 × 72	0·28 ÷ 72

E2 A large bottle of a chemical is emptied out into beakers, and fills $12\frac{1}{2}$ beakers. A full beaker holds 450 millilitres of chemical.

Which of these calculations gives the total amount of chemical in the bottle to start with? (Do not use a calculator.)

$$12\cdot5 \div 450 \qquad 12\cdot5 \times 450 \qquad 450 \div 12\cdot5 \qquad 450 - 12\cdot5$$

E3 16 people share out some money equally between them. Each person gets £5·45. How much was shared out?

E4 The entry fee to Heartbreak House went up from £1·30 to £1·45. In the week before the increase, 7532 people visited the house. In the week after, the number was 6653.

(a) How much money was paid altogether by visitors in the week before the increase?

(b) How much was paid altogether in the week after the increase?

(c) Was it a good idea to increase the entry fee?

E5 Blagdon Town Football Club needs £165 to buy new shirts. A firm gives the club 750 badges to sell.

(a) How much should the club charge for each badge, if they want to raise £165 by selling them all?

(b) What should they charge for each badge if they expect to sell only 500 badges?

E6 1 metre of metal tube weighs 0·72 kg and costs £1·08.
(a) What does 5·5 metres of tube weigh?
(b) What does 5·5 metres of tube cost?

E7 A metal tube 6·5 metres long costs £6·41. How much does 1 metre cost, to the nearest penny?

E8 (a) Calculate the cost per metre of each of these hoses, to the nearest penny.

(b) Which hose is better value?

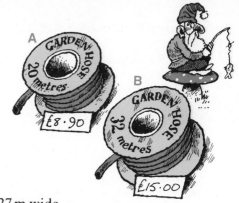

E9 A rectangular field is 42 m long and 27 m wide. The owner wants to put up a fence round the edge of the field, leaving one gap 2 m wide.

(a) How many metres of fencing does he need?

(b) If the fencing costs £4·65 per metre, how much will he have to pay?

E10 Here are two carpets, A and B.

(a) Calculate the area of carpet A, in square metres (m²).

(b) Calculate the cost of 1 m² of carpet A.

(c) Calculate the cost of 1 m² of carpet B.

(d) Which carpet is more expensive per square metre?

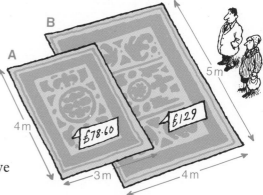

E11

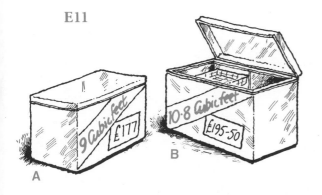

Here are two freezers.

(a) How much do you pay for each cubic foot of storage in freezer A? (Round off to the nearest penny.)

(b) How much do you pay for each cubic foot in freezer B?

(c) Which freezer is better value for money?

E12 (a) The return fare from London to Paris is £46. How much is that in French francs, if £1 is worth 10·75 francs? Round off your answer to the nearest franc.

(b) The fare goes up to £49·50. What is the new fare in francs, to the nearest franc?

9 Flow charts

A Rules

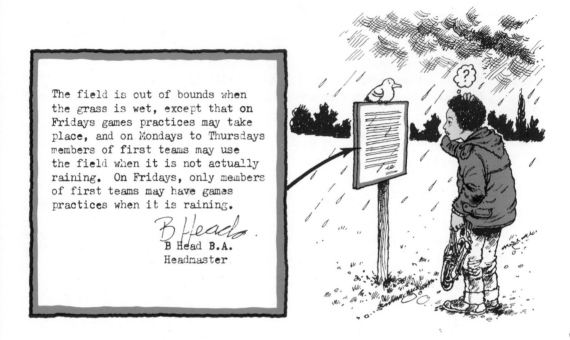

The field is out of bounds when the grass is wet, except that on Fridays games practices may take place, and on Mondays to Thursdays members of first teams may use the field when it is not actually raining. On Fridays, only members of first teams may have games practices when it is raining.

B Head B.A.
Headmaster

Look at the rules for using the field.
Use them to answer these questions.

A1 On Wednesday the grass is wet, but it is not raining. You want to have a games practice but you are not a member of a first team. Can you use the field?

A2 It is raining on Thursday. You are in the first team but you do not want a games practice.
Can you use the field?

A3 On Friday the grass is wet. It is not raining. You are not a member of a first team but you want a games practice.
Can you use the field?

A4 On Monday it is dry. You want a games practice. You are not in a first team.
Can you use the field?

Rules are often difficult to understand. It is easier to answer questions 'yes' or 'no' than to follow complicated rules.

One way of doing this is to use a **flow chart**.

Here is a flow chart for the same rules as before. It tells you when you can and cannot use the field.

You answer each question 'yes' or 'no', and follow the lines. The last box you get to tells you whether you can use the field or not.

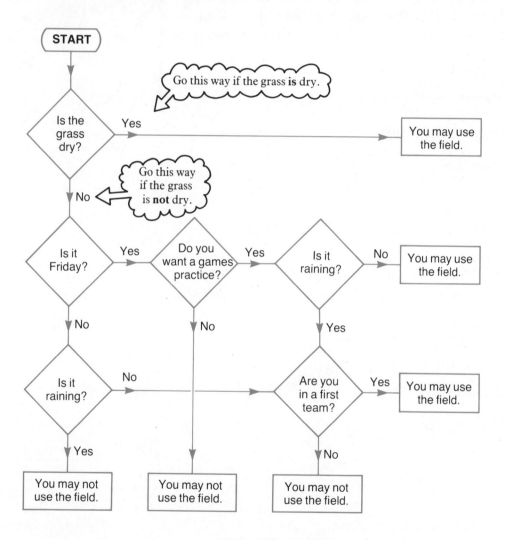

A5 It is Tuesday. The grass is wet, but it is not raining. You are in a first team. Can you use the field?

A6 It is Friday and it is raining. You want a games practice but you are not in a first team. Can you use the field?

On the school tennis courts you can play singles or doubles.
You can play either at lunchtime or after school.

Here are the rules for using the courts.

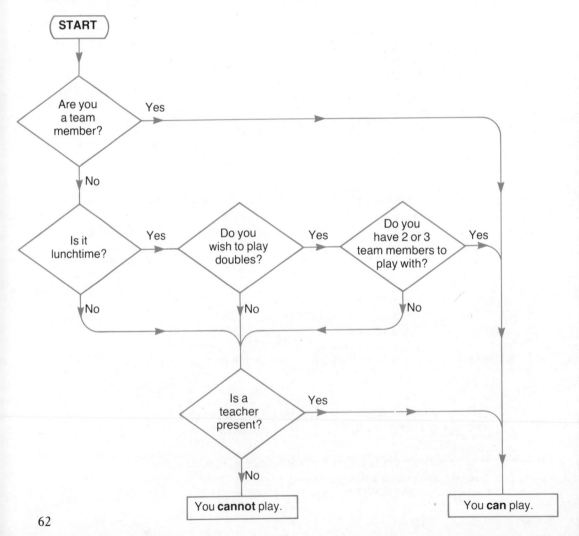

'Team members may use the courts at any time.
Non-team members may play only if a teacher
is present, except that at lunchtime they may
play doubles if at least 2 of the 4 players are
team members. After school, a teacher must be
present for any doubles matches involving
non-team members.

Here are the same rules written as a flow chart.

START

Are you a team member? — **Yes** →

↓ **No**

Is it lunchtime? — **Yes** → Do you wish to play doubles? — **Yes** → Do you have 2 or 3 team members to play with? — **Yes** →

↓ **No** ↓ **No** ↓ **No**

Is a teacher present? — **Yes** →

↓ **No**

You **cannot** play.

You **can** play.

Use either the rules or the flow chart to answer questions A7 to A11.

A7 You are not a team member. You want to play singles with a team member at lunchtime. There is no teacher present. Can you play?

A8 It is Tuesday after school. You want to play doubles with three team members. You are not a team member yourself. There is no teacher present. Can you play?

A9 You are a team member. You and another team member want to play singles after school. There is no teacher available. Can you play?

A10 Two of you who are not team members want to play doubles with two team members. It is lunchtime, and there is a teacher present. Can you play?

A11 You are not a team member. Do you need a teacher if you want to play singles with a team member at lunchtime?

A12 Was it easier to use the rules or the flow chart to answer questions A7 to A11?

A13 This flow chart gives the rules for using the school minibus.

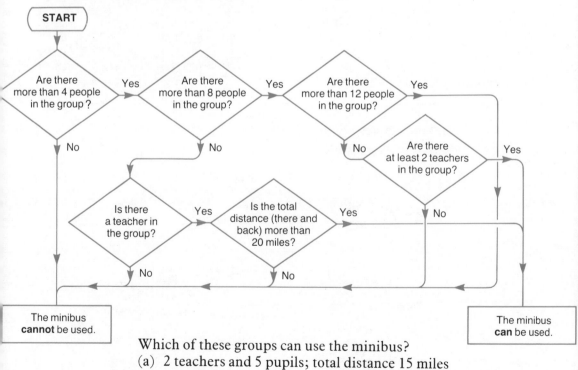

Which of these groups can use the minibus?
(a) 2 teachers and 5 pupils; total distance 15 miles
(b) 1 teacher and 4 pupils; total distance 25 miles
(c) 1 teacher and 8 pupils; total distance 40 miles

B Sorting

B1 At Boffin Bay you can catch six kinds of fish.
The Boffin Bay Council has made a flow chart. It helps fishermen who want to know what kind of fish they have caught.

The coloured boxes tell you the name of the fish.

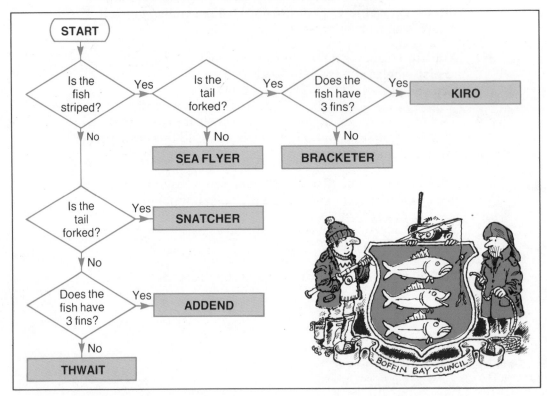

What kinds of fish are these?
Tails don't count as fins!

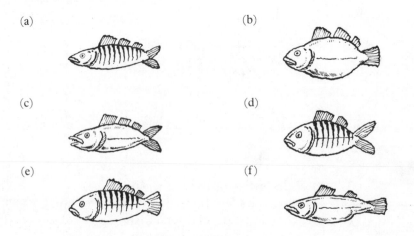

(a)

(b)

(c)

(d)

(e)

(f)

B2 The flow diagram below is for identifying types of yacht.
It works for most, but not all, ocean-going single-hulled yachts.

You need to know the names
of various parts of a yacht,
shown in the diagram on the right.

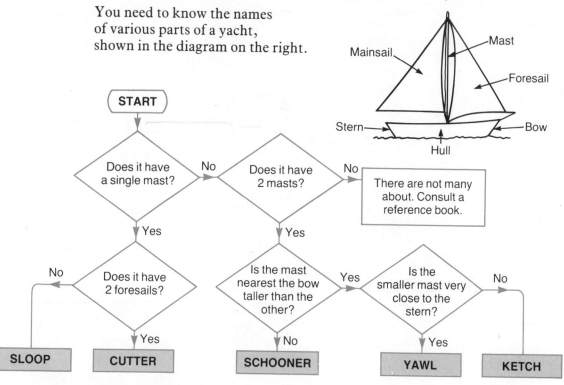

What kinds of yacht are these?

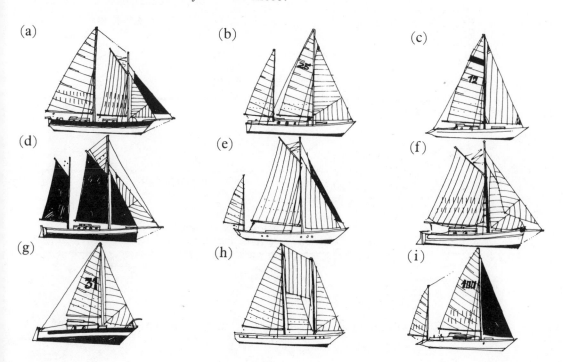

(a)

(b)

(c)

(d)

(e)

(f)

(g)

(h)

(i)

C Number flow charts

C1 (a) Draw two columns, and head them A and B. Now follow the instructions in this flow chart.

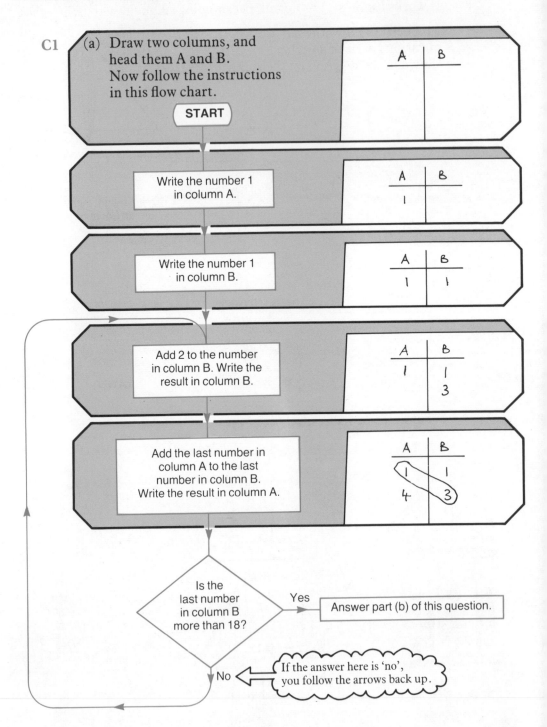

START

Write the number 1 in column A.

Write the number 1 in column B.

Add 2 to the number in column B. Write the result in column B.

Add the last number in column A to the last number in column B. Write the result in column A.

Is the last number in column B more than 18?

Yes → Answer part (b) of this question.

If the answer here is 'no', you follow the arrows back up.

No

(b) What is special about the numbers in column A?

C2 (a) Follow the instructions in this flow chart, but starting with the number 40.

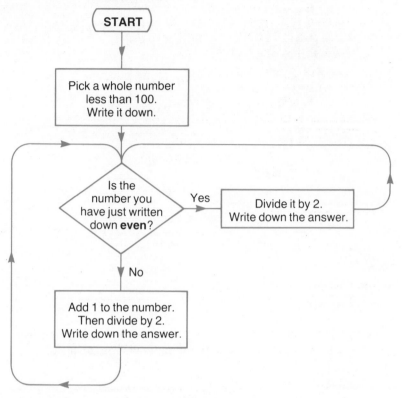

(b) Pick three numbers of your own.
Follow the flow chart for each one.

(c) What number do you always get to in the end?

(d) If you do **exactly** what is in the flow chart, would you ever stop? Why not?

(e) How could you change the flow chart so that you do stop?

C3 (a) Follow the instructions in this flow chart, but starting with the number 5.

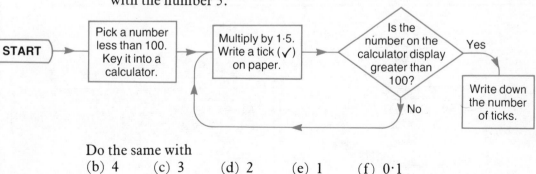

Do the same with
(b) 4   (c) 3   (d) 2   (e) 1   (f) 0·1

D A robot

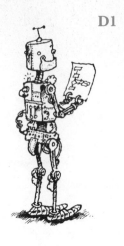

D1 This robot is going to test a flow chart for crossing a road.

It will only do exactly what the flow chart tells it to do.

Here is the flow chart.

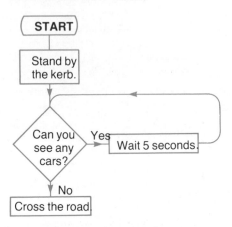

Each picture below tells you that there is something wrong with the flow chart. Write down what is wrong with the flow chart for each one.

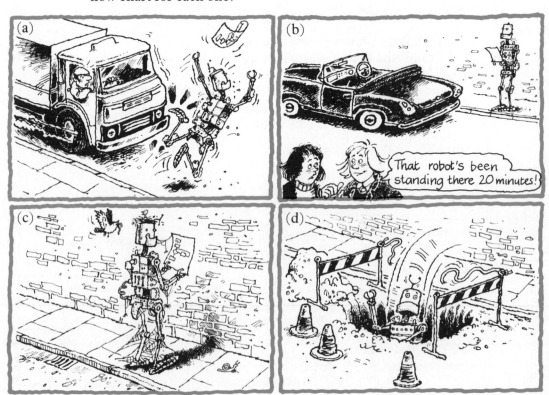

Review 2

6 Multiplication

6.1 Do not use a calculator.

$$38\cdot4 \times 0\cdot73 = 51\cdot302$$

   (a) How can you tell straight away that this calculation must be wrong?

Which of these calculations must be wrong?

(b) $65\cdot2 \times 1\cdot08 = 63\cdot446$ (c) $9\cdot64 \times 0\cdot85 = 8\cdot194$
(d) $3\cdot85 \times 0\cdot08 = 24\cdot712$ (e) $0\cdot984 \times 75 = 82\cdot316$
(f) $4\cdot08 \times 2\cdot73 = 0\cdot8644$ (g) $0\cdot86 \times 0\cdot95 = 0\cdot817$

6.2 Do not use a calculator.
Choose which of the four numbers is closest to the answer to each calculation.

(a) $3\cdot2 \times 5\cdot1$	12	15	18	21
(b) $6\cdot8 \times 4\cdot9$	30	35	40	45
(c) $0\cdot93 \times 8\cdot76$	4	6	8	10
(d) $52 \times 0\cdot48$	25	35	45	55

6.3 Do not use a calculator.
Write down a rough answer for each of these.

   (a) $8\cdot2 \times 4\cdot1$ (b) $7\cdot7 \times 3\cdot9$ (c) $2\cdot89 \times 4\cdot07$
   (d) $5\cdot86 \times 3\cdot92$ (e) $8\cdot03 \times 7\cdot15$ (f) $2\cdot34 \times 6\cdot88$
   (g) $31\cdot5 \times 2\cdot98$ (h) $61\cdot3 \times 4\cdot08$ (i) $48\cdot9 \times 2\cdot78$

6.4 A car used $9\cdot3$ gallons of petrol on a journey to Scotland. If the cost of petrol was £1·84 a gallon, how much did the petrol for the journey cost (to the nearest penny)?

6.5 A $0\cdot55$ kW greenhouse heater was left on for 72 hours.

   (a) How many units of electricity did it use?
      (Number of units = power in kW × time in hours)

   (b) If the cost of electricity was £0·05 per unit, how much did it cost to leave the heater on?

6.6 Some curtain material costs £3·80 a metre.
Tape for edging it costs £0·68 a metre.

Is this bill correct? If not, write out a correct bill.

6·6m of curtain material	£ 25·80
3·5m of tape	£ 23·80
Total	£ 49·60

7 Investigations

7.1 In this kind of number chain, you add the 1st and 2nd numbers to get the 3rd, and the 2nd and 3rd to get the 4th, and so on.

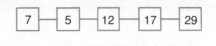

(a) Continue the chain which starts with 3, 4 until you have eight numbers altogether.

(b) Find the missing numbers in the chain below. Describe how you did it, step by step.

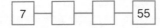

8 Division

8.1 Without using a calculator, say whether the answers to these are greater than 1 or less than 1.

(a) $43 \cdot 6 \div 7 \cdot 2$ (b) $0 \cdot 95 \div 8 \cdot 4$ (c) $15 \cdot 3 \div 68 \cdot 9$

(d) $4 \div 800$ (e) $41 \cdot 5 \div 41 \cdot 4$ (f) $1 \cdot 635 \div 7 \cdot 01$

8.2 14 sheets of plywood have a total thickness of $9 \cdot 1$ cm. How thick is each sheet? Check by multiplying.

8.3 A table costs £54·50, but if you buy it together with a set of 4 chairs, the total cost is £125.

(a) How much do you pay for the set of 4 chairs?

(b) How much do you pay for each chair, to the nearest penny?

8.4 Hameed got this receipt for some petrol and oil he bought.

(a) How much did the petrol cost per litre?

(b) How much did the oil cost per litre?

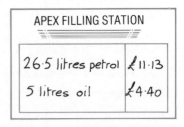

8.5 (a) 13 people shared some money equally, and each person got £5·20. How much was shared out?

(b) If the same amount is shared equally between 12 people, how much will each person get, to the nearest penny?

8.6 (a) Calculate the cost per kg of the cat litter in each of these bags. Round off each answer to the nearest penny.

(b) Which bag is better value?

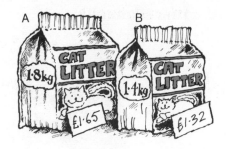

9 Flow charts

9.1 (a) Follow the instructions in this flow chart, starting with the number 3.

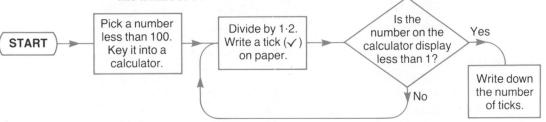

(b) Do the same, starting with (i) 40 (ii) 45 (iii) 50.

(c) Suppose the third box in the flow diagram said 'Divide by 0·2' and you started with 50. What would happen?

9.2 This is a flow chart for sorting screws into four boxes A, B, C and D.

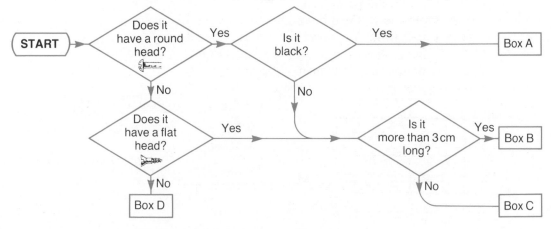

Here are some screws, all drawn full size. Which box does each screw go in?

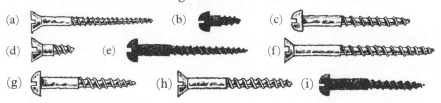

71

M Miscellaneous

M1 If £1 is worth $1·35 (1·35 dollars) and $1 is worth £0·74, write down the missing prices in the pictures below.

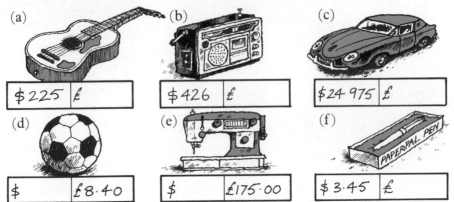

(a) $225 £

(b) $426 £

(c) $24 975 £

(d) $ £8·40

(e) $ £175·00

(f) $3·45 £

M2 1 inch is equal to 2·54 cm.
Curtain material is 48 inches wide. What is this in centimetres, to the nearest centimetre?

M3 A chemist weighs out 500 grams of tablets, and counts the tablets. There are 830 tablets.
How much does each tablet weigh? Round off your answer to the nearest tenth of a gram.

M4 A 2·5-litre tin of paint costs £3·95.
(a) Work out the cost per litre.
(b) 1 litre of the paint will cover 7 square metres.
What is the cost of painting 1 square metre? Round off your answer to the nearest penny.

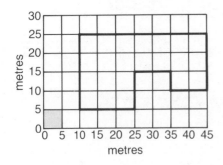

M5 This is the ground plan of a large house.

(a) What area is represented by the shaded square?

(b) What is the area of the ground plan of the house?

M6 Work these out without using a calculator.

(a) 40×30 (b) 50×50 (c) 600×20

(d) 60×50 (e) $20 \times 20 \times 20$ (f) 300×300

M7 This mileage chart gives the distances by road between various cities in Britain.

For example, the distance between Edinburgh and Newcastle is 106 miles.

Mileage chart
Distances in miles by road

Birmingham	Bristol	Cardiff	Edinburgh	Glasgow	Leeds	Liverpool	Manchester	Newcastle	London
87									
102	43								
286	365	368							
287	365	370	44						
109	194	208	191	210					
90	160	164	210	212	73				
79	159	172	210	211	40	35			
200	284	298	106	143	91	153	128		
110	116	153	373	392	190	197	184	273	

(a) How far is it from Leeds to Bristol?
(b) How far is it from Leeds to Newcastle?
(c) Which city on the chart is furthest from Leeds?
(d) Which city is furthest from Cardiff?
(e) Which two cities are closest together?
(f) Which two are furthest apart?
(g) Calculate the total length in miles of this round trip:
London → Bristol → Manchester → Leeds → London.

M8

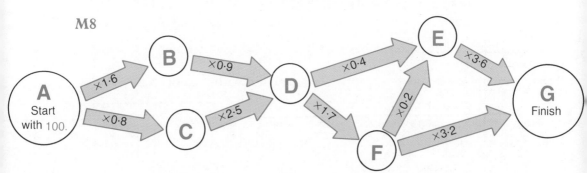

This is a calculator 'maze'. If you start with 100 at A and go A→B→D→E→G, you do $100 \times 1.6 \times 0.9 \times 0.4 \times 3.6 = \mathbf{207.36}$.

Start at A with 100.
(a) Find out which route from A to G gives the largest answer at G. Write down the answer and the route.

(b) Find which route gives the smallest answer.

10 Patterns (2)

A Repeating patterns: reflection symmetry

This is part of an endless **repeating pattern**. You can think of the
pattern as going on and on in exactly the same way in both directions.

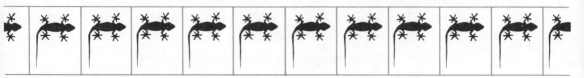

The lizard is called the **repeating unit** of the pattern.

If we reflect the lizard like this,

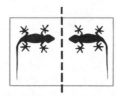

we can use the lizard and its reflection together as a single repeating
unit. We get this pattern:

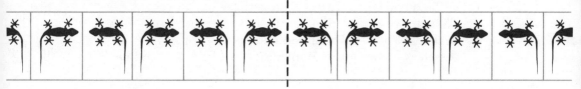

The dotted line on the pattern above is a line of reflection symmetry
of the **whole pattern**.
The diagram below shows how every lizard pairs off with its reflection.

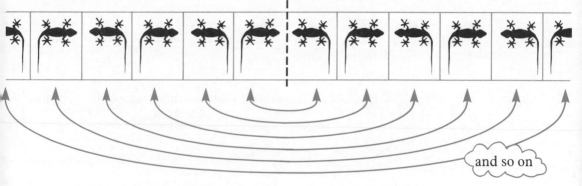

and so on

There are many other lines of reflection symmetry of the pattern
at the bottom of the previous page.
Two of them are shown below. (Remember that the pattern
goes on and on in both directions.)

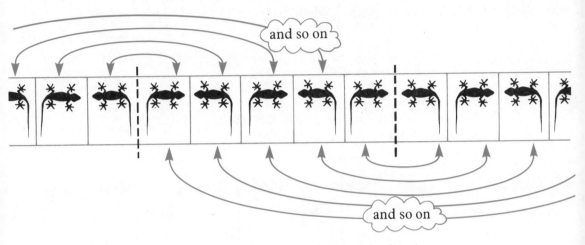

Notice how the lizards pair off on either side of a line of reflection symmetry.
Each lizard pairs off with its reflection.

A1 (a) Is the line marked A a line of reflection symmetry of the
pattern below? (See if the lizards pair off properly
either side of A.)

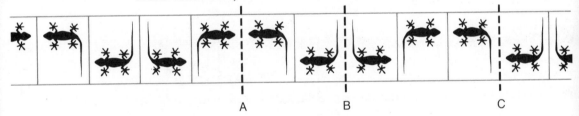

(b) Is line B a line of reflection symmetry of the pattern?
(See if the lizards pair off properly either side of B.)

(c) Is line C a line of reflection symmetry of the pattern?

A2 Is line P a line of reflection symmetry of the pattern below?
(Do the lizards pair off properly either side of P?)

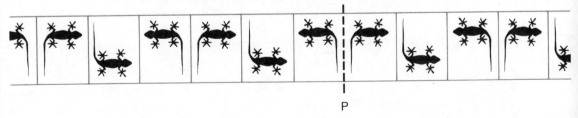

A3 Which of the lines marked P, Q, R are lines of reflection symmetry of this repeating pattern?

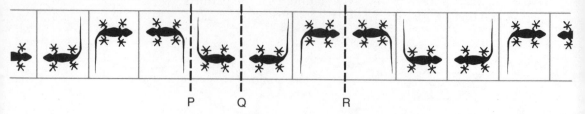

A4 Which of the lines marked A, B, C are lines of reflection symmetry of this repeating pattern?

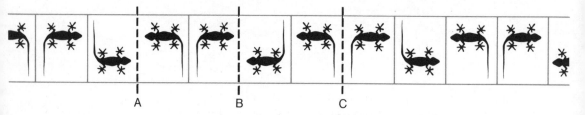

A5 Here are some more repeating patterns.
For each one, write down which of the marked lines are lines of reflection symmetry.

(a)

(b)

(c)

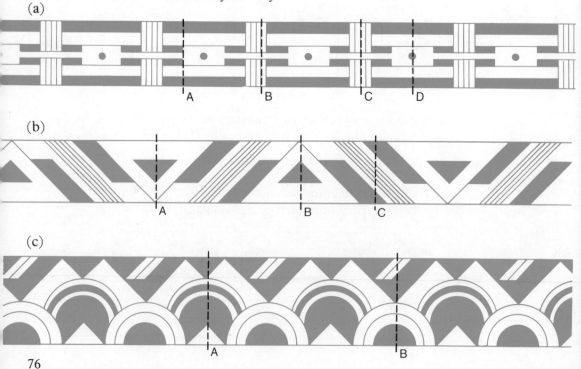

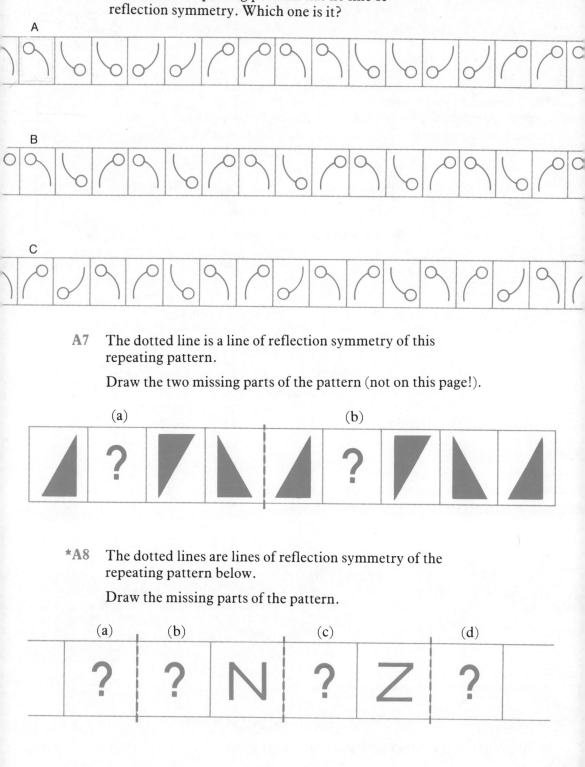

A6 One of these repeating patterns has no line of reflection symmetry. Which one is it?

A

B

C

A7 The dotted line is a line of reflection symmetry of this repeating pattern.

Draw the two missing parts of the pattern (not on this page!).

(a)   (b)

*A8 The dotted lines are lines of reflection symmetry of the repeating pattern below.

Draw the missing parts of the pattern.

(a)   (b)   (c)   (d)

B Repeating patterns: 2-fold rotation centres

Here again is the lizard which was used to make the first pattern on page 74.

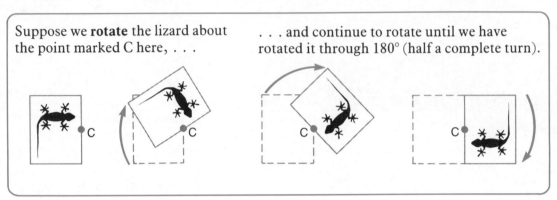

Suppose we **rotate** the lizard about the point marked C here, . . .

. . . and continue to rotate until we have rotated it through 180° (half a complete turn).

The original lizard and the rotated one together look like this.

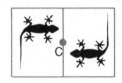

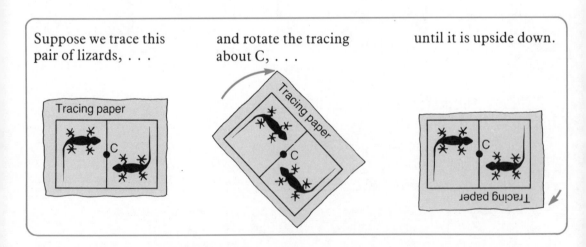

Suppose we trace this pair of lizards, . . .

and rotate the tracing about C, . . .

until it is upside down.

There are 2 positions where the tracing fits the pair of lizards.

So the point C is the **2-fold rotation centre** of the pair of lizards.

We can use the pair of lizards as a repeating unit.
Here is the pattern we get.

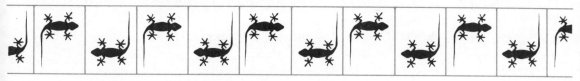

A simplified drawing of this pattern is printed on worksheet B1–3.

You need worksheet B1–3 and tracing paper.

B1 Put your tracing paper over
the pattern on the worksheet.
Trace the pattern.

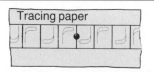

Keep the tracing in position.
Put a sharp point on the dot
marked A.

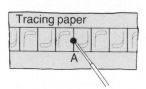

Rotate the tracing about A
until it is upside down.

You will find that the tracing
fits the pattern again.
(Remember that the pattern is
supposed to go on and on.)

This shows that **A is a 2-fold
rotation centre of the whole pattern**.

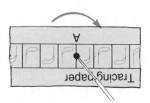

Now start again with the tracing in its original position.
This time rotate the tracing about the point B.

You should find that B is a 2-fold rotation centre of the pattern.

Mark the other 2-fold rotation centres of the same pattern on
the worksheet, using the symbol ● .

B2 There are four other repeating patterns on the worksheet.
Three of them have 2-fold rotation centres. One of them does not.

Find as many 2-fold rotation centres as you can, for each pattern.
Mark them on the worksheet, using the symbol ● .

C Making repeating patterns with a stencil

You need one of the special stencils and a fairly large sheet of paper.

Each stencil can be used to draw four pictures. For example, the
'F-stencil' can be used to draw these four pictures.
(To get the rectangle we draw round the outside edge of the stencil.)

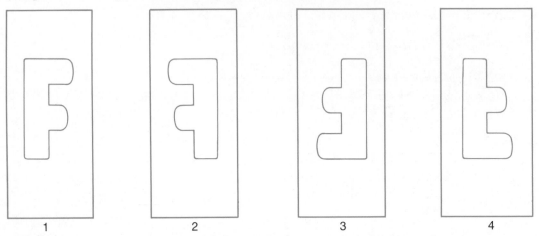

We can make a very simple kind of repeating pattern by repeating just one
of these four pictures. For example, by repeating picture 2, we get this.

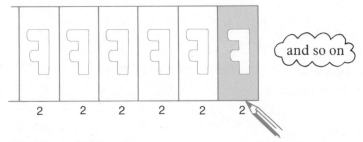

and so on

**By drawing round the rectangle each time we make sure that the
pictures are equally spaced.**

The repeating unit in the pattern above consists of the single picture 2.
The pattern below goes 2 4 2 4 2 4 2 4 . . .
The repeating unit is 2 4 (or 4 2).

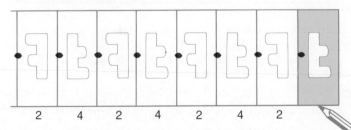

This pattern has 2-fold rotation centres as shown here.

80

C1 Start by drawing the four different pictures you can make with your stencil. Number them from 1 to 4.

For example:

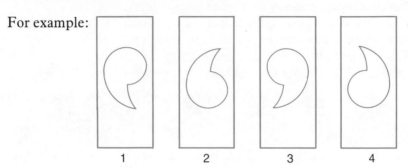

1   2   3   4

Choose a repeating unit made up of **two** of the pictures.
For example, 32:

3   2

Now draw as much as you can of the repeating pattern using the repeating unit you have chosen.
For example, the repeating unit 32 above would give this pattern:

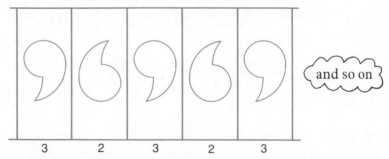

and so on

3 2 3 2 3

Draw on your pattern the lines of reflection symmetry (if any) and the 2-fold rotation centres (if any) of the pattern.

C2 Use the same set of four pictures as in question C1.
This time choose a repeating unit made up of the four pictures in some order, for example 2431.

Draw as much as you can of the repeating pattern and mark its lines of reflection symmetry (if any) and 2-fold rotation centres (if any).

C3 Repeat question C2, but with the four pictures in a different order.

D The period of a repeating pattern

Suppose we choose any point A on a repeating pattern.
We look along the pattern to find the first time this point repeats exactly.
Call the 'first repeat' A′.

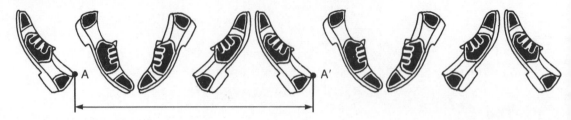

The distance from A to A′ is called the **period** of the repeating pattern.

> **D1** Measure the period, in centimetres, of the repeating pattern shown above.

> **D2** Measure the periods of each of these repeating patterns.

(a)

(b)

(c)

(d)

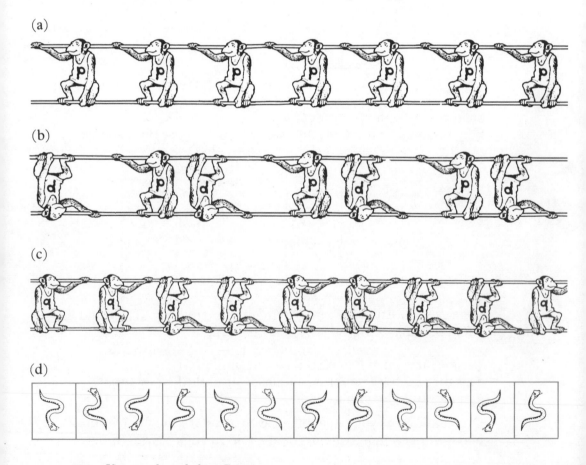

> **D3** *You need worksheet B1–4.*

82

11 Negative numbers

A Temperatures below zero

Negative numbers are used for temperatures below freezing point.
$^-2°C$ means 2 degrees C below zero.

Suppose the temperature starts at $^-2°C$ and then rises by 5 degrees.
Afterwards it will be 3°C. (Check this on the scale below.)

We can write an addition to show what happens to the temperature.

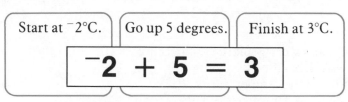

| Start at $^-2°C$. | Go up 5 degrees. | Finish at 3°C. |

$$^-2 + 5 = 3$$

A1 At 6 a.m. the temperature in Murmansk is $^-7°C$.
By 9 a.m. it has risen by 12 degrees.

(a) What is the temperature at 9 a.m.?

(b) Copy and complete this addition sum for the temperature.

$$^-7 + \ldots = \ldots$$

A2 Write an addition sum for each of these.
(a) The temperature starts at $^-4°C$ and rises by 6 degrees.
(b) The temperature starts at $^-7°C$ and rises by 2 degrees.
(c) The temperature starts at $^-1°C$ and rises by 9 degrees.
(d) The temperature starts at $^-6°C$ and rises by 6 degrees.

A3 Copy and complete each of these.

(a) $^-5 + 1 = \ldots$ (b) $^-12 + 15 = \ldots$ (c) $^-8 + 6 = \ldots$ (d) $^-3 + 8 = \ldots$

A4 The temperature at Aviemore rises from $^-3°C$ at dawn
to 10°C at noon.
(a) By how many degrees has it risen?
(b) Copy and complete this addition sum for the temperature.

$$^-3 + \ldots = 10$$

A5 Suppose the temperature goes up from $^-4°C$ to 3°C.
(a) By how many degrees has it risen?
(b) Copy and complete this addition.

$$^-4 + \ldots = 3$$

A6 Copy and complete each of these.

(a) $^-6 + \ldots = ^-1$ (b) $^-3 + \ldots = 8$
(c) $^-4 + \ldots = 0$ (d) $^-7 + \ldots = ^-2$

Suppose the temperature starts at 5°C and then **falls** by 7 degrees.
Afterwards it will be $^-2$°C. (Check this on the scale.)

We can write a **subtraction** to show what happens.

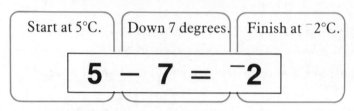

Start at 5°C.   Down 7 degrees.   Finish at $^-2$°C.

$$5 - 7 = ^-2$$

A7 At noon in Vladivostok the temperature is 10°C.
By dusk it has fallen by 15 degrees.
(a) What is the temperature at dusk?
(b) Copy and complete this subtraction.

$10 - 15 = \ldots$

A8 Next day at noon it is $^-1$°C. By dusk it has fallen by 20 degrees.
(a) What is the temperature at dusk?
(b) Copy and complete this subtraction.

$^-1 - 20 = \ldots$

A9 Copy and complete each of these.

(a) $2 - 9 = \ldots$ (b) $^-4 - 2 = \ldots$ (c) $^-6 - 5 = \ldots$ (d) $^-1 - 1 = \ldots$

A10 The temperature falls from 3°C to $^-6$°C.
(a) By how many degrees does it fall?
(b) Copy and complete this subtraction.

$3 - \ldots = ^-6$

A11 Write an addition or a subtraction for each of these.

(a) The temperature at Glencoe is $^-4$°C. It then rises by 12 degrees.

(b) In Moscow it is $^-20$°C. Later in the day it is $^-5$°C.

(c) At noon in New York it is 8°C. By dusk it is $^-5$°C.

(d) At dawn in Antarctica it is $^-35$°C. At noon it is $^-28$°C.

A12 Write temperature 'stories' (like those in question A11) for
each of these.

(a) $^-10 + 18 = 8$ (b) $5 - 18 = ^-13$

B Temperature graphs

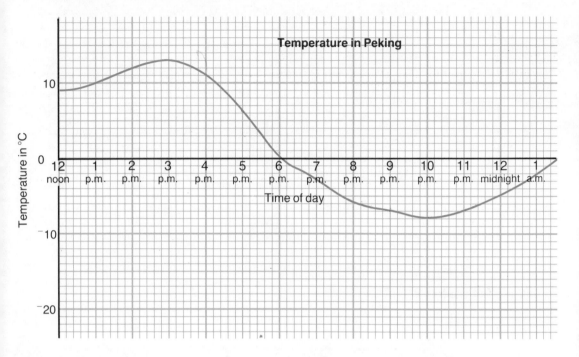

Temperature in Peking

The graph shows that the temperature in Peking at 8 p.m. was ⁻6°C.
By 10 p.m. the temperature had fallen to ⁻8°C.

From ⁻6°C to ⁻8°C is a fall of 2 degrees. We can write this subtraction.

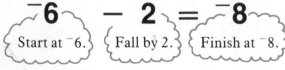

$$^-6 \quad - \quad 2 \quad = \quad ^-8$$

Start at ⁻6.   Fall by 2.   Finish at ⁻8.

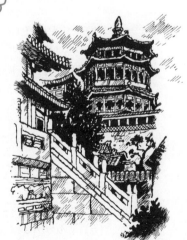

B1 (a) What was the temperature at 7 p.m.?

(b) What was it at 9 p.m.?

(c) Write a subtraction similar to the one above for the change in temperature between 7 p.m. and 9 p.m.

B2 (a) What was the temperature at 5 p.m.?

(b) What was it at 8 p.m.?

(c) Write a subtraction for the change in temperature between 5 p.m. and 8 p.m.

B3 In which hour of the day did the biggest fall in temperature happen? (Was it between 3 p.m. and 4 p.m., or between 4 p.m. and 5 p.m., etc.?)

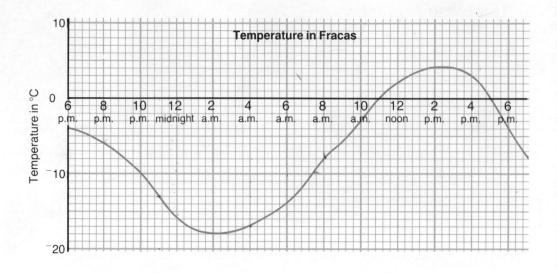

Temperature in Fracas

On this graph, the temperature at 10 a.m. was ‾3°C.
By noon it had risen to 2°C.

This was a rise of 5 degrees. We can write this addition.

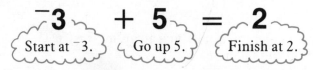

$$^-3 \quad + \quad 5 \quad = \quad 2$$

Start at ‾3.   Go up 5.   Finish at 2.

B4 (a) What was the temperature in Fracas at 8 a.m.?
(b) What was it at 10 a.m.?
(c) Write an addition, similar to the one above, for
the change in temperature between 8 a.m. and 10 a.m.

B5 Write an addition or subtraction showing how the temperature
changes between

(a) 8 p.m. and midnight   (b) 6 a.m. and 10 a.m.
(c) 8 a.m. and 2 p.m.   (d) 2 p.m. and 6 p.m.

B6 The temperature at 4 a.m. was ‾17°C.
Some time later it had risen by 9 degrees.

(a) What time was it then?
(b) Copy and complete: ‾17 + 9 = . . .

B7 (a) What was the temperature at 11 p.m.?
(b) What was it at 7 a.m.?

B8 When was the temperature ‾16°C?

B9 For how many hours was the temperature above zero?

C The skating contest

At the Minors' Skating Contest,
the judges give points.

When the judges like a skater,
they give scores like 4 or 6.

When the judges do not like a
skater, they can give negative scores.

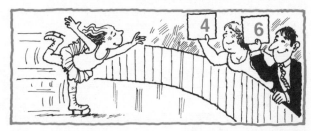

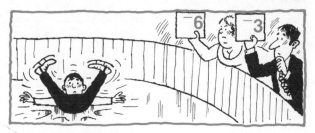

The judges' scores are added up.
Sometimes the judges disagree with one another!

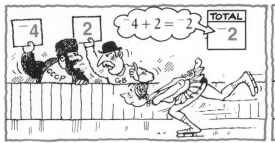

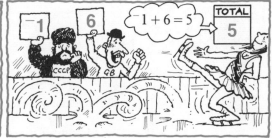

C1 Find the total score in each of these pictures.

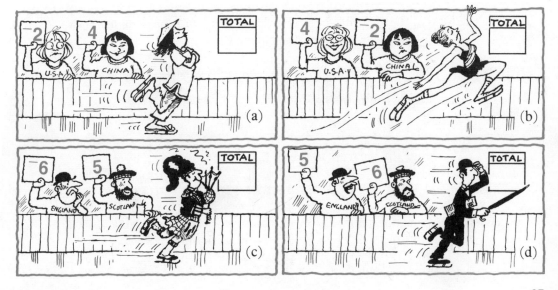

You can total up the points by thinking of the number line.
For 3 points, move 3 to the **right**. For ⁻3 points, move 3 to the **left**.
Start at 0.

Here are some examples.

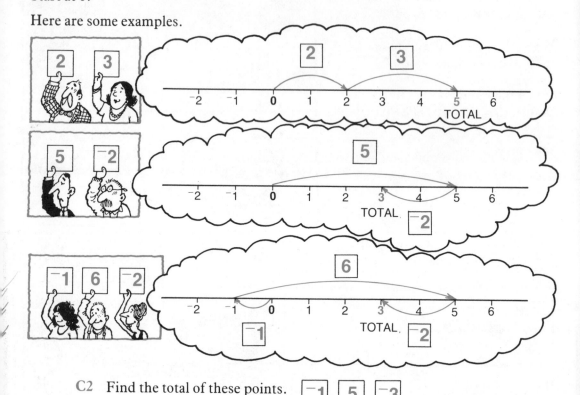

C2 Find the total of these points. ⁻1 5 ⁻3

C3 Find the total of each of these sets of points.
(a) ⁻1, ⁻2, 5   (b) 1, ⁻1, 3, ⁻4, ⁻1, ⁻1   (c) ⁻1, ⁻1, ⁻3, 8, 2
(d) 3, 2, ⁻6, ⁻2, 8   (e) 0, ⁻4, ⁻3, 1, 1   (f) ⁻6, 2, 7, ⁻3

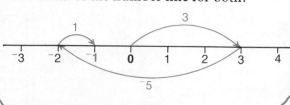

Finding the total of these points 3 ⁻5 1
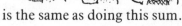
is the same as doing this sum.
$3 + ⁻5 + 1 =$

You think of the number line for both.

C4 Work out the answers to these.
(a) $2 + ⁻5 + 4 =$ (b) $⁻3 + ⁻4 + ⁻5 =$ (c) $3 + ⁻3 + 4 + 1 =$
(d) $⁻1 + 1 + ⁻4 + 0 =$ (e) $3 + ⁻9 + 12 + ⁻5 =$ (f) $⁻2 + ⁻3 + ⁻4 + ⁻5 =$

C5 (a) Work out $5 + ⁻2$.   (b) Now work out $5 - 2$.
      (c) Work out $7 + ⁻3$.   (d) Now work out $7 - 3$.
      (e) Work out $2 + ⁻4$.   (f) Now work out $2 - 4$.
      (g) Work out $⁻1 + ⁻5$.   (h) Now work out $⁻1 - 5$.

Look at your answers to question C5. You should have found that the answers to (a) and (b) are the same: (a) $5 + {}^-2 = 3$ (b) $5 - 2 = 3$
Adding ${}^-2$ is the same as subtracting 2.

The answers to (c) and (d) are the same. So are the answers to (e) and (f) and the answers to (g) and (h).

Adding ${}^-3$ is the same as subtracting 3.
Adding ${}^-4$ is the same as subtracting 4, and so on.

So, for example, $8 + {}^-2$ is the same as $8 - 2$,
$\qquad\qquad\quad {}^-6 - 3$ is the same as ${}^-6 + {}^-3$.

C6　Find the answers to these. Use the method you think is easiest.

(a) $6 + {}^-5$ (b) $4 + {}^-3$ (c) ${}^-5 - 7$ (d) ${}^-3 - 4$
(e) $6 + {}^-2$ (f) ${}^-3 + {}^-1$ (g) $17 + {}^-9$ (h) ${}^-10 - 3$
(i) $9 - 12$ (j) $7 + {}^-2$ (k) ${}^-1 + {}^-8$ (l) $4 + {}^-7$

Marks

This is a game for two players. You need a dice and two counters. (Coins will do.)

START
YOU START WITH 0

Volunteer for job because you like music.
$+\boxed{1}$

Made to move school piano.
$+\boxed{{}^-2}$

Arrive early for school.
Add $\boxed{2}$
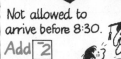

Answer card found.
$-\boxed{6}$

Not allowed to arrive before 8:30.
Add $\boxed{{}^-2}$
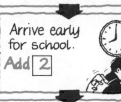

Get full marks in maths test.
$+\boxed{3}$

Put your counters on START.

You take turns to roll the dice. Move your counter forward the number of places shown on the dice.

Add or subtract the marks you get to your total. Keep a record of your total on paper.

The game ends either when a player has a total of 10 marks (Teacher's pet!) or when a player gets a total of ${}^-10$ marks. (Bottom of the class!)

You have all your books ready for Monday.
$+\boxed{1}$
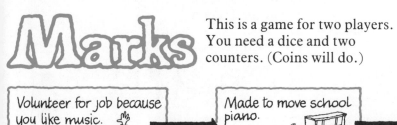

Team loses 114 – 0.
Subtract $\boxed{3}$

It is Tuesday.
$+\boxed{{}^-3}$
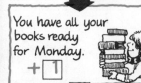

Chosen for school team.
Add $\boxed{4}$

Cat dies.
Add $\boxed{{}^-3}$
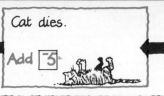

Feed caretaker's cat.
$+\boxed{2}$
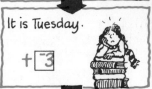

*D Subtracting negative numbers

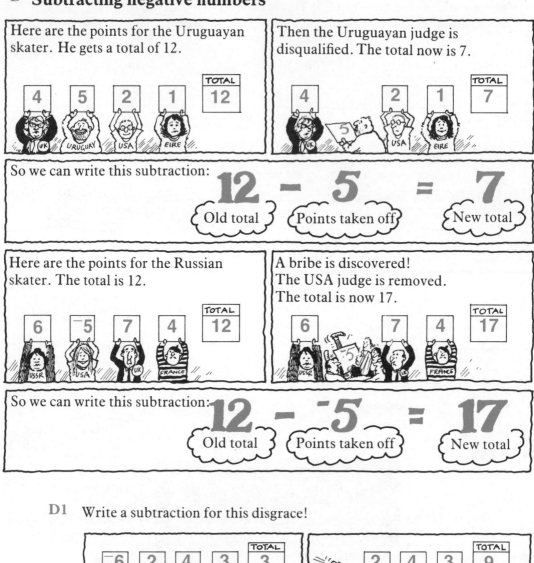

Here are the points for the Uruguayan skater. He gets a total of 12.

TOTAL 12

4 5 2 1

Then the Uruguayan judge is disqualified. The total now is 7.

TOTAL 7

4 2 1

So we can write this subtraction:

12 – 5 = 7

Old total — Points taken off — New total

Here are the points for the Russian skater. The total is 12.

TOTAL 12

6 ⁻5 7 4

A bribe is discovered!
The USA judge is removed.
The total is now 17.

TOTAL 17

6 7 4

So we can write this subtraction:

12 – ⁻5 = 17

Old total — Points taken off — New total

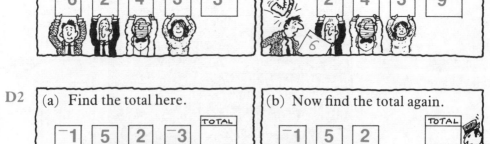

D1 Write a subtraction for this disgrace!

⁻6 2 4 3 **TOTAL 3**

2 4 3 **TOTAL 9**

D2 (a) Find the total here.

⁻1 5 2 ⁻3 **TOTAL**

(b) Now find the total again.

⁻1 5 2 **TOTAL**

(c) Write a subtraction for the totals.

D3 (a) Find the total here.

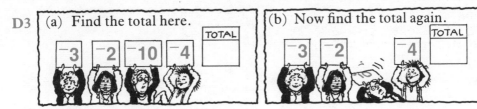

(b) Now find the total again.

(c) Write a subtraction for the totals.

D4 The French skater has a total of 8.
After a protest, a score of ⁻4 is taken off.

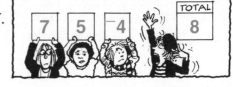

(a) What is the new total?

(b) Write a subtraction for this.

D5 (a) Find the total of these scores: 3, 4, ⁻2, ⁻5, 1
(b) Now find the total without the ⁻5.
(c) Write a subtraction for this.

D6 (a) Find the total of 2, 7, ⁻4, 1 and ⁻1.
(b) Now find the total without the ⁻4.
(c) Write a subtraction for this.

D7 (a) Find the total of ⁻3, ⁻1, 2 and ⁻5.
(b) Now find the total without the ⁻5.
(c) Write a subtraction for this.

D8 Here are the scores for the Maltese skater.

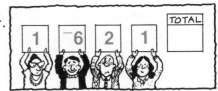

(a) What is the total?
(b) What is the new total if the ⁻6 is taken off?
(c) Write a subtraction for this.

D9 The New Zealand skater scores 2, ⁻3, ⁻4, 1 and 0.
(a) What is her total?
(b) What is her new total if the ⁻4 is taken off?
(c) Write a subtraction for this.

D10 Here are the Italian skater's scores.

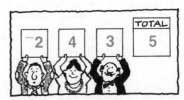

Which of these is better?

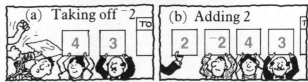

(a) Taking off ⁻2

(b) Adding 2

Taking off a score of $^-2$ ... $5 - {}^-2 = 7$

is the same as adding 2. $5 + 2 = 7$

Subtracting $^-2$ is the same as adding 2.
Subtracting $^-3$ is the same as adding 3.
Subtracting $^-4$ is the same as adding 4, and so on.

So $6 - {}^-3$ is the same as $6 + 3 = 9$,
and $^-4 - {}^-2$ is the same as $^-4 + 2 = {}^-2$.

D11 Copy and complete these.

(a) $6 - {}^-1$
$= 6 + 1$
$=$

(b) $^-3 - {}^-5$
$= {}^-3 + 5$
$=$

(c) $^-2 - {}^-1$
$= {}^-2 + 1$
$=$

(d) $10 - {}^-8$
$= 10 + 8$
$=$

(e) $6 - {}^-4$
$=$
$=$

(f) $^-5 - {}^-5$
$=$
$=$

(g) $7 - {}^-4$
$=$
$=$

(h) $^-3 - {}^-6$
$=$
$=$

(i) $^-4 - {}^-1$
$=$
$=$

D12 Find the answers to these.
(a) $^-6 - {}^-2$ (b) $4 - {}^-1$ (c) $^-10 - {}^-2$ (d) $^-8 - {}^-3$
(e) $6 - {}^-10$ (f) $^-6 - {}^-10$ (g) $0 - {}^-4$ (h) $^-1 - {}^-1$
(i) $^-4 - {}^-3$ (j) $2 - {}^-5$ (k) $7 - {}^-3$ (l) $^-2 - {}^-8$

D13 (a) What do you get when you subtract $^-3$ from 6?
(b) What do you get when you subtract $^-2$ from $^-3$?

D14 You have a total of $^-10$.
A score of $^-6$ is taken off.
What is your total now?

D15 What is the new total when a score of $^-8$ is taken off
a total of 4?

D16 In some of these you have to subtract a negative number.
In others you have to subtract an ordinary number.
(a) $5 - {}^-1$ (b) $5 - 1$ (c) $^-2 - 4$ (d) $^-2 - {}^-4$
(e) $6 - {}^-3$ (f) $^-6 - {}^-3$ (g) $^-2 - {}^-5$ (h) $1 - 7$
(i) $12 - 8$ (j) $^-12 - {}^-4$ (k) $0 - 6$ (l) $0 - {}^-6$

D17 These are a mixture of additions and subtractions. Be careful!

(a) 2 + $^-$5   (b) 2 − $^-$5   (c) 5 + $^-$2   (d) 5 − $^-$2

(e) $^-$3 + $^-$6   (f) $^-$4 − 5   (g) 2 + $^-$7   (h) 3 − $^-$8

(i) $^-$9 − $^-$2   (j) 10 + $^-$8   (k) 10 − 12   (l) $^-$2 − $^-$6

*E Negative numbers on a calculator

Some calculators can handle negative numbers and some cannot.

Those which can, have a 'change sign' key, usually labelled $\boxed{+\!/\!-}$.

To key in $^-$5, you press $\boxed{5}\boxed{+\!/\!-}$.

The $\boxed{+\!/\!-}$ comes **after** the number.

To do $^-$5 − $^-$9, you press $\boxed{5}\boxed{+\!/\!-}\boxed{-}\boxed{9}\boxed{+\!/\!-}\boxed{=}$.

You will need a calculator with a 'change sign' key for these questions.

E1 (a) Without using a calculator, work out 5 − $^-$3.

(b) Now use a calculator to work out 5 − $^-$3, and check that the answer is the same.

E2 Do each of these without using a calculator, and then use the calculator to check them.

(a) 4 + $^-$9   (b) $^-$3 + $^-$8   (c) $^-$10 − $^-$3   (d) 5 − $^-$8

(e) $^-$2 − $^-$2   (f) 4 − $^-$8   (g) $^-$8 + $^-$9   (h) 0 − $^-$6

E3 Key in a number. Then press the 'change sign' key twice. What happens?

E4 The temperature difference between the inside and the outside of a building is given by the formula

Temperature difference = temperature inside − temperature outside

Calculate the temperature difference in each of these cases.

(a) Temperature inside: 23·0 °C. Temperature outside: 18·5 °C.

(b) Temperature inside: 15·3 °C. Temperature outside: $^-$4·4 °C.

(c) Temperature inside: $^-$2·8 °C. Temperature outside: $^-$10·3 °C.

(d) Temperature inside: $^-$7·2 °C. Temperature outside: $^-$1·8 °C.

(e) Why is the answer to part (d) a negative number?

12 Formulas and graphs

A Springs

Jane is doing an experiment. She hangs a spring
from the table and puts weights on the end of it.
Then she measures how high the end of the spring is
above the floor.

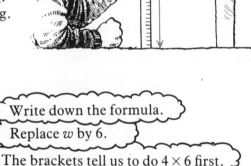

She has worked out a formula for the height of the
end of the spring above the floor. It is

$$h = 40 - (4 \times w).$$

h is the height, in cm, of the end of the spring.
w is the weight, in kg, on the end of the spring.

Suppose Jane puts 6 kg on the spring.
This means that $w = 6$.
So you can work out h like this.

$h = 40 - (4 \times w)$	Write down the formula.
$h = 40 - (4 \times 6)$	Replace w by 6.
$h = 40 - 24$	The brackets tell us to do 4×6 first.
$h = 16$	

So the end of the spring is 16 cm above the floor.

A1 Use the formula $h = 40 - (4 \times w)$ to work out h when $w = 2$.
Write out your working as above.

A2 Jane hangs 8 kg on the spring.
What is the height of the end above the floor?

A3 What will the height be if Jane hangs 5 kg on the spring?

A4 (a) Work out h when $w = 3$.
(b) Work out h when $w = 9$.

A5 Work out the height of the end of the spring when the
weight on the end is
(a) 4 kg   (b) 1 kg   (c) 7 kg   (d) $\frac{1}{2}$ kg

A6 How high is the end of the spring when there is $5\frac{1}{2}$ kg
on the end of it?

94

Rajesh hangs the spring from a different table.
He has worked out a formula for the height of the end
of the spring.
He writes it like this.

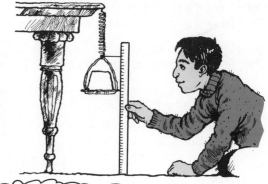

The formula is
$$h = 34 - (w \times 4)$$
h is the height in cm above the floor
w is the weight in kg

He works out h when w = 6 like this.

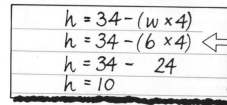

$h = 34 - (w \times 4)$
$h = 34 - (6 \times 4)$
$h = 34 - 24$
$h = 10$

Replace w by 6, and
work out the brackets first.

A7   (a) Copy the formula for Rajesh's spring.
     (b) Work out h when he puts 4 kg on the spring.
          Write out the working as above.

A8   What is the height of the end of Rajesh's spring when he puts
     2 kg on it?

A9   Work out h when w is
     (a) 3   (b) 5   (c) 7   (d) 8   (e) 1

A10 (a) What is h when $w = \frac{1}{2}$?
     (b) What is h when $w = \frac{1}{4}$?

A11 When Rajesh hangs no weight from the spring, then $w = 0$.
     Work out h when $w = 0$.

A12 Work out h when $w = 9$. Explain what the answer means.

A13 Work out the height of the end of the spring for each of these weights.

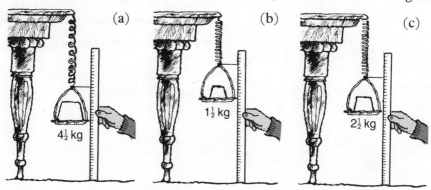

(a)   (b)   (c)

$4\frac{1}{2}$ kg $1\frac{1}{2}$ kg $2\frac{1}{2}$ kg

95

B Shorthand

There is a shorthand we can use.
Instead of $4 \times w$ or $w \times 4$ we write $4w$.

Notice we write $4w$ instead of $4 \times w$ **or** $w \times 4$.
People do **not** write $w4$ instead of $w \times 4$.

Jane's formula was $h = 40 - (4 \times w)$.

We can write it $h = 40 - 4w$.

Rajesh's formula was $h = 34 - (w \times 4)$.

We write it $h = 34 - 4w$.

We leave out the brackets.
In a formula without brackets, we always
do any multiplying first.

B1 Write these formulas using the shorthand.
     (a) $h = 50 - (6 \times w)$ (b) $h = 100 - (10 \times w)$ (c) $h = 160 + (w \times 5)$
     (d) $a = (6 \times b) + (c \times 5)$ (e) $y = (x \times 5) + (z \times 10)$ (f) $c = (a \times 4) - (3 \times b)$

Here is a formula written the short way: $h = 160 - 5w$.
Suppose $w = 10$. You work out h like this.

$$h = 160 - 5w$$
$$\text{When } w = 10 \quad h = 160 - 5 \times 10$$
$$h = 160 - 50$$
$$h = 110$$

Write the formula.

Replace w by 10.
$5w$ means 5×10.

Multiply first.

B2 Use the formula $h = 160 - 5w$ to find h when $w = 6$.
     Write out the working as above.

B3 Copy and complete this working
     to find h when $w = 4$.

$$h = 160 - 5w$$
$$\text{When } w = 4, \quad h = 160 - 5 \times 4$$

B4 Use the formula $h = 160 - 5w$ to find h when w is
     (a) 8   (b) 5   (c) 1   (d) 0

B5 Use the formula $h = 100 - 6w$ to find h when w is
     (a) 10   (b) 8   (c) 9   (d) 4

B6 Use the formula $r = 5s + 10$ to find r when
     (a) $s = 6$ (b) $s = 10$ (c) $s = 5$ (d) $s = 1$

B7 If $y = 6x - 12$, find y when
(a) $x = 3$ (b) $x = 5$ (c) $x = 2$ (d) $x = 10$

B8 If $t = 8s + 9$, find t when
(a) $s = 6$ (b) $s = 0$ (c) $s = 10$ (d) $s = 1$

B9 (a) Write $p = 95 + (q \times 5)$ the short way.
(b) Find p when $q = 6$.
(c) Find p when $q = 10$.
(d) What is p if q is 3?

If $q = 3$, we sometimes say the **value** of q is 3.

B10 Use the formula $t = 9j - 10$ to find the value of t when the value of j is 3.

B11 If $r = 100 + 5s - 4t$, find the value of r when
(a) $s = 4$ and $t = 1$ (b) $s = 6$ and $t = 2$ (c) $s = 10$ and $t = 10$
(d) $s = 0$ and $t = 6$ (e) $s = 0$ and $t = 0$ (f) $s = 3$ and $t = 2$

B12 Trains run from Dumbella to Beulah.
The time taken for the whole journey depends on the number of
stations the train stops at on the way.

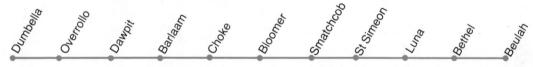

The formula for the journey time is $t = 27 + 2n$.
t is the journey time in minutes.
n is the number of stations the train stops at (not counting
the ends of the line).

(a) Find t when n is 5.
(b) How long will it take to get from Dumbella to Beulah if the
train stops at
(i) Dawpit and Bloomer
(ii) Barlaam, Choke and Smatchcob
(iii) Overrollo, Dawpit, Bloomer, St Simeon and Bethel
(iv) every station
(c) How long will it take if the train goes non-stop from
Dumbella to Beulah?

B13 City Printing Services print posters for discos, concerts, and so on.
They supply posters in packs of fifty. The cost depends on the
number of packs ordered. The formula for the cost is $C = 25 + 4n$.
C is the cost in pounds; n is the number of packs ordered.

(a) Find C when $n = 6$. (b) Find C when $n = 4$.
(c) Find the cost of 15 packs of posters.

C Drawing graphs for formulas

Here is a formula for the height of the end of a spring above the floor.

$$h = 50 - 8w$$

h stands for the height, in cm, of the end of the spring.
w stands for the weight, in kg, on the end.

We can use the formula to find h when w is 0, 1, 2, 3 and so on.
When we have done this we can show the values of w and h in a table.

w	0	1	2	3	4	5	6
h	50	42	34	26	18	10	2

Now we can plot these values on a graph.
We decide what scales to use for w and h.
Then we plot the points.

The points are in a straight line. It makes sense to draw the line
through them.

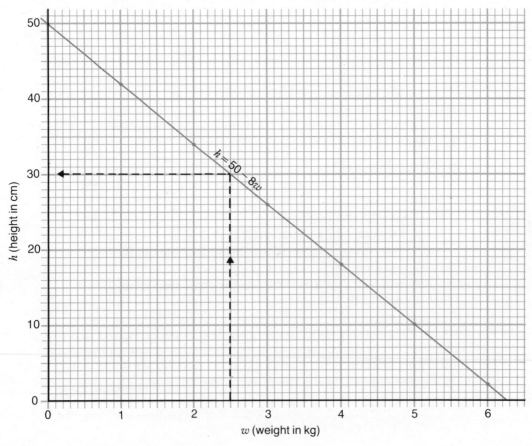

We can use the graph to find h for any value of w.
For example, when $w = 2\cdot5$, we see that $h = 30$.

C1 Use the graph to find h when $w = 4\cdot5$.
Use a ruler or your finger to follow the lines.

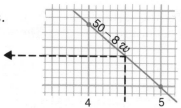

C2 Use the graph to find h when $w = 1\cdot5$.

C3 Use the graph to find h when   (a) $w = 3\cdot5$ (b) $w = 0\cdot5$ (c) $w = 5\cdot5$

C4 I hang $1\cdot5$ kg on the spring. How high is the end above the floor?

C5 How high is the end of the spring from the floor, when the weight on the end is
(a) $2\cdot5$ kg   (b) $3\cdot5$ kg   (c) $0\cdot4$ kg   (d) $1\cdot6$ kg

C6 What is the value of w when   (a) $h = 25$ (b) $h = 0$

C7 For a different spring the formula is $h = 80 - 10w$.
h stands for the height, in cm, of the end of the spring.
w stands for the weight, in kg, on the end.

(a) Copy and complete this table. Work out h for each value of w.

w	0	1	2	3	4	5	6	7	8
h				50					10

When $w = 7$, $h = 80 - 10 \times 7$
$= 80 - 70$
$= 10$

(b) Draw axes like these on graph paper.
Plot the points from your table.
Draw a straight line through them.
Write the formula along the line.
(c) Use your graph to find the value of h when $w = 3\cdot5$.
(d) Find h when $w = 6\cdot5$.
(e) Find h when $w = 7\cdot2$.
(f) What is h if w is $1\cdot8$?
(g) What is h if w is $2\cdot8$?
(h) I hang $5\cdot8$ kg on the spring.
How high is the end above the floor?
(i) What weight do I need to put on the spring to make the height of the end 36 cm above the floor?

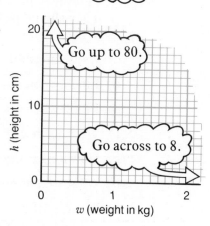

When you hang a weight on a spring, the spring stretches.

Let l stand for the length of the spring, in cm.
Let w stand for the weight on it, in kg.

For the spring in the picture there is a formula connecting l and w.
The formula is $l = 20 + 5w$.

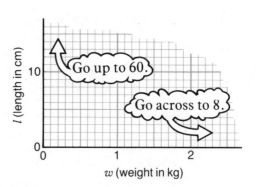

C8 In the picture, $w = 5$.
Use the formula $l = 20 + 5w$ to work out l
when $w = 5$. Check from the picture that your
answer is correct.

C9 (a) Copy and complete this table showing values of w and l.

w	0	1	2	3	4	5	6	7	8
l						45			

(b) Draw axes like these
on graph paper.

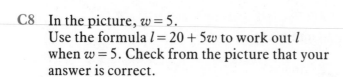

Plot the points from your table.
They should be in a straight line. Draw the line through them.
Write the formula along the line.

(c) Use your graph to find l when $w = 4 \cdot 6$.

(d) Find l when $w = 0 \cdot 8$.

(e) Find l when $w = 2 \cdot 6$.

(f) What value of w makes $l = 36$?

(g) How long is the spring if I hang $1 \cdot 2$ kg on it?

(h) What weight must I hang on the spring to make it 52 cm long?

(i) What is l if $w = 7 \cdot 2$?

(j) What is w if $l = 39$?

C10 A different spring has the formula $l = 14 + 3w$.

(a) Copy and complete this table.

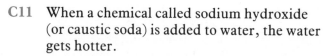

w	0	1	2	3	4	5	6
l							

(b) Draw axes on graph paper, with w **across** from 0 to 6 and l **up** from 0 to 40.
Plot the points from your table and draw the graph.

(c) From your graph find l when $w = 2\cdot7$.

(d) Find w when $l = 18$.

C11 When a chemical called sodium hydroxide (or caustic soda) is added to water, the water gets hotter.

The formula for the temperature of the water in this tank is

$$t = 24 + 8m.$$

t is the temperature, in degrees C.
m is the amount of sodium hydroxide added, in kg.

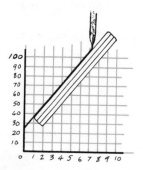

(a) Copy and complete this table showing values of m and t.

m	0	1	2	3	4	5	6	7
t	24							

(b) Draw axes on graph paper, with m across from 0 to 10, and t up from 0 to 100.

Plot the points from your table, and join them up.

(c) Use your graph to find t when $m = 2\cdot5$.

(d) How much sodium hydroxide is needed to make the temperature of the water 76 °C?

(e) What will the temperature be if $1\cdot5$ kg of sodium hydroxide is put in the water?

(f) Use a ruler to extend your graph to the right.
What is t when $m = 8\cdot5$?

(g) What value of m makes $t = 100$?
Check by putting this value of m into the formula.

(h) Why is it not sensible to extend the graph further than where $t = 100$?

101

D More shorthand

The ground clearance of a car or lorry
is the distance between the bottom of the
car or lorry and the ground.

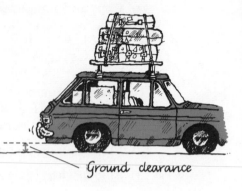

For the car in the picture there is a formula
for the ground clearance. It is

$$g = 40 - (w \div 10).$$

g is the ground clearance, in cm.
w is the load on the car, in kg.

Ground clearance

There is a shorthand for $w \div 10$.

We write $\dfrac{w}{10}$ instead of $w \div 10$.

So the formula becomes $g = 40 - \dfrac{w}{10}$.

We can leave out the brackets.
We do the dividing first.

This is how to find the ground clearance when $w = 260$.

$$g = 40 - \frac{w}{10}$$

When $w = 260$, $\quad g = 40 - \dfrac{260}{10}$

$$g = 40 - 26$$
$$g = 14$$

Write the formula.

Replace w by 260.

Do the division first.

D1 Use the formula to find g when $w = 200$.
Write the working as shown above.

D2 Use the formula to find g when $w = 150$.

D3 What is g when $w = 100$?

D4 What is the ground clearance of the car when it is not
carrying any load?

D5 Work out the value of g when w is
(a) 350 (b) 50 (c) 80 (d) 110

D6 Copy and complete this table showing values of w and g.

w	0	50	100	150	200	250	300	350	400
g									

D7 (a) Draw axes like these on graph paper.
Plot the values of w and g from
your table for question D6.

Draw the straight line through the
points.

(b) Use your graph to find g when $w = 180$.

(c) What is g when $w = 360$?

(d) What value of w makes $g = 0$?
What happens to the car then?

(e) When the ground clearance is 12 cm,
what load is the car carrying?
Use your graph to find out.

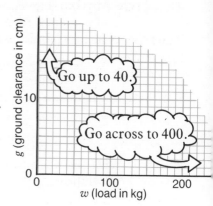

D8 For this van, the formula for the ground clearance is

$$g = 50 - \frac{w}{20}.$$

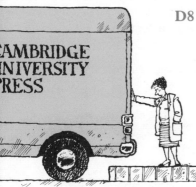

(a) Find g when $w = 200$.
(b) Find g when $w = 360$.
(c) What is the ground clearance when the van
carries a load of 600 kg?
(d) The van is carrying a load of 500 kg.
Can it reverse over a kerb 15 cm high?
Explain how you get your answer.
(e) What happens to the van when it carries a load
of 1000 kg?

D9 The picture on the right shows a jack
for lifting cars.

The height of the jack depends on
the number of turns of the handle.

The formula is $h = \dfrac{n}{5} + 30$.

h is the height, in cm.
n is the number of turns.

(a) Find h when $n = 20$, like this.

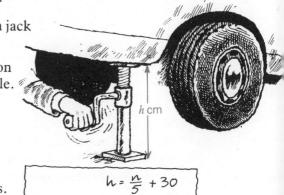

$$h = \frac{n}{5} + 30$$
When $n = 20$, $h = \frac{20}{5} + 30$
$$=$$

Find h when n is   (b) 30   (c) 25   (d) 15   (e) 0   (f) 1

D10 Write these formulas the short way.
(a) $y = (x \div 3) - 2$ (b) $p = 7 + (q \div 4)$ (c) $e = (f \div 3) + 17$

D11 At ground level, water boils at 100°C.
The temperature at which water boils is
called its 'boiling point'.

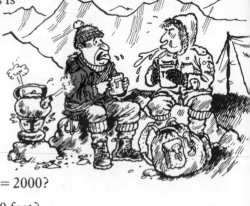

As you go up a mountain, the boiling
point changes.
The formula for the boiling point is

$$b = 100 - \frac{h}{1000}.$$

b is the boiling point, in degrees C.
h is the height, in feet.

(a) What is the boiling point when $h = 2000$?

(b) What is the boiling point at 10 000 feet?

(c) Ben Nevis is about 4000 feet high.
What is the boiling point of water on top of Ben Nevis?

(d) Mount Everest is about 30 000 feet high.
What is the boiling point of water on top of Mount Everest?

D12 As you go deeper into the Earth, it gets hotter.
The temperature in this mineshaft is given
by the formula

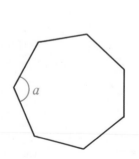

$$t = 15 + \frac{d}{100}.$$

t is the temperature, in degrees C.
d is the depth, in metres, below the surface.

(a) What is t when $d = 600$?

(b) What is the temperature 1000 m below the surface?

(c) What is the temperature 2000 m below the surface?

(d) The deepest part of the mine is 3500 m deep.
How hot is it there?

D13 The size of one of the angles of a regular polygon
depends on the number of sides the polygon has.

The formula for the angle is

$$a = 180 - \frac{360}{n}. \qquad \overleftarrow{\text{360 divided by } n.}$$

a is the angle, in degrees.
n is the number of sides.

(a) Use the formula to find a when n is 6.
(b) What is a when n is 10?
(c) What is the size of each angle in a regular polygon
with 20 sides?

10 Patterns (2)

10.1 Which of the lines a, b, c, d are lines of reflection symmetry of this endless repeating pattern?

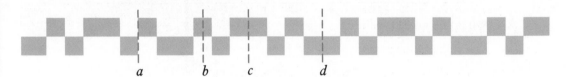

10.2 Which of the points A, B, C, D are 2-fold rotation centres of this endless repeating pattern?

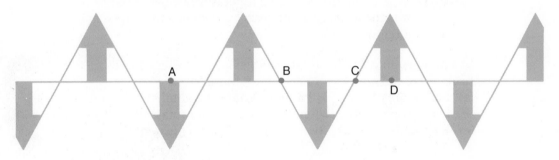

10.3 This is part of an endless repeating pattern, but one picture is missing.
The dotted lines are all lines of reflection symmetry of the pattern.
Draw the missing picture.

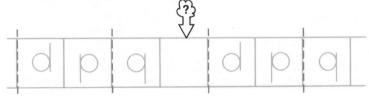

11 Negative numbers

11.1 (a) If the temperature falls from 12 °C to ⁻8 °C, by how many degrees does it fall?
(b) Copy and complete this subtraction: $12 - \ldots = {}^-8$.

11.2 Work these out.
(a) $^-5 + 2$ (b) $^-7 + 9$ (c) $^-3 - 4$ (d) $2 - 6$ (e) $^-8 + 3$

11.3 This graph shows the temperature in a northern town during a day in winter.

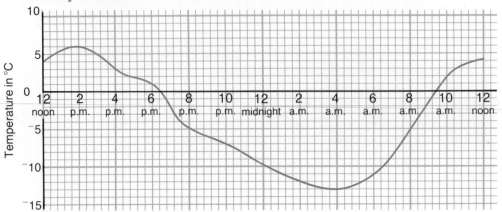

(a) Use the graph to find the temperature at   (i) 4 p.m. (ii) 5 a.m.
(b) For how many hours was the temperature below $^-5\,°C$?
(c) What was the difference, in degrees, between the lowest and highest temperatures?

11.4 In a diving contest there are five judges.
Each judge can give a score between $^-5$ and 5.
(a) Sam scores 2, $^-1$, $^-3$, 1 and 0. What is his total?
(b) Joan scores 3, 4, $^-2$, 1 and $^-1$. What is her total?
(c) Ken scores $^-2$, $^-3$, $^-5$, $^-1$ and $^-4$. What is his total?

11.5 Work these out.
(a) $3 + ^-1$ (b) $^-2 + ^-4$ (c) $^-3 + ^-2$ (d) $4 + ^-5$ (e) $2 + ^-7$

12 Formulas and graphs

12.1 Use the formula $q = 60 - 4p$ to find q when p is
(a) 2   (b) 10   (c) 8   (d) 0   (e) 15

12.2 Use the formula $b = 3a - 7$ to find b when a is
(a) 4   (b) 5   (c) 9   (d) 3   (e) 20

12.3 Use the formula $s = \dfrac{r}{5} + 12$ to find s when r is
(a) 20   (b) 100   (c) 5   (d) 15   (e) 0

12.4 Use the formula $d = 28 - \dfrac{c}{4}$ to find d when c is
(a) 12   (b) 20   (c) 0   (d) 28   (e) 4

12.5 The cost of a journey in one of Tiny's Taxis is given by the formula $C = 40 + 50d$.
C is the cost in pence and d is the number of miles.

(a) How much does it cost to travel 2 miles?
(b) How much does it cost to travel 5 miles?

12.6

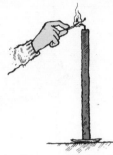

Hema lights a candle.
The formula for its height
afterwards is

$$h = 30 - 4t.$$

h is the height in cm.
t is the time the candle
has been burning, in hours.

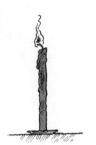

(a) Copy and complete this table showing values of t and h.

t	0	1	2	3	4	5	6	7
h								

(b) Draw axes like these on graph paper.
Plot the points from your table,
and draw the line through them.

(c) Use the graph to find the height
of the candle $3\frac{1}{2}$ hours after
it was lit.

(d) When was the candle 20 cm high?
(How many hours after being lit?)

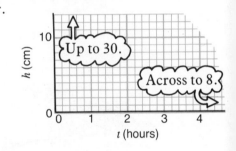

(e) How long did the candle take to burn down completely?

(f) What is t when h is 12?

M Miscellaneous

M1 This map shows a wood.
Each grid square which is more
than half covered by the wood
has a tree drawn in it.

(a) What area (in km²) does
one grid square represent?

(b) Estimate the area of
the wood.

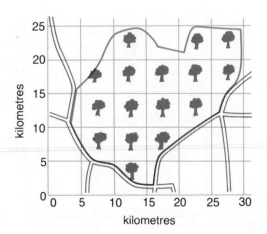

M2 Round off
(a) 6 637 492 to the nearest million
(b) 6 637 492 to the nearest thousand
(c) 4·6836 to 2 decimal places
(d) 6·194 to 1 decimal place
(e) 0·597 to 2 decimal places

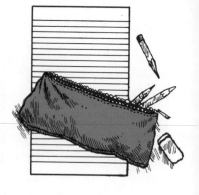

M3 A sheet of paper has 26 lines ruled on it, with equal spaces between them.

(a) How many spaces are there?

(b) The distance between the top and bottom lines is 17 cm.
How big is the space between each line and the one below it?

M4 (a) 13 people share £426 equally between them.
How much does each person get, to the nearest penny?

(b) 18 people share out some money equally. Each person gets £3·60. How much was shared out?

M5 Which of these tubes of toothpaste is better value?
Explain why.

A   B

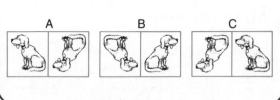

M6
When you reflect this design in the dotted line. . . . . . which of these do you see?

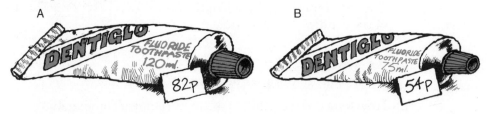

M7
When you turn this design upside down . . . . . . which of these do you see?

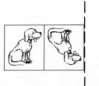
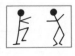
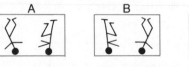
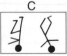

The questions in this section are based on the work in these booklets
(or chapters in *Book BT*): *Views*, *Speed 1* and *Volume*.

A Views

You need two matchboxes.

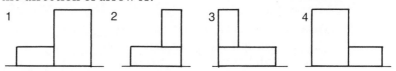

A1 Put the two matchboxes on the table
as shown in the picture on the right.

  (a) Which of the diagrams below shows
the view you see when you look in
the direction of arrow A?

  (b) Draw the view looking in the direction of arrow B.

  (c) Draw a plan view of the matchboxes (looking down from
directly above them).

A2 Put the two matchboxes in
this position.

  (a) Draw views in the directions
A, B, C and D.

  (b) Draw a plan.

A3 Here is a model church.

Four of the diagrams below
are views of the model.
The others are not.

Which **are** views of the model,
and which direction were they
taken from?

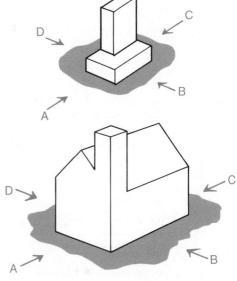

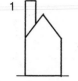
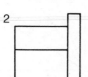
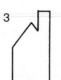
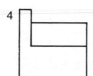
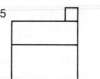
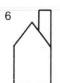

B Speed

B1 Three girls are running a race.
This picture shows them some time after the race started.
The scale shows how far they are from the start, in metres.

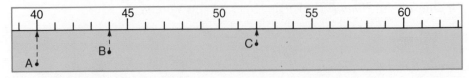

Here are the girls 1 second later.

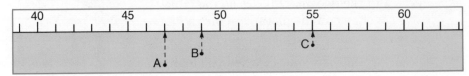

(a) How far did A run in that 1 second?
(b) Write down A's speed for that second.
(c) Write down B's speed for that second.
(d) Write down C's speed for that second.
(e) Who ran fastest during that second?

B2 How far do you go in 8 seconds at a constant speed of 5 m/s?

B3 If you go at a constant speed of 6 m/s how far do you go in
(a) 2 seconds   (b) 5 seconds   (c) 10 seconds   (d) 7 seconds

B4 A train is going at a constant speed of 65 m/s.
How far does it go in 8 seconds?

B5 Three cyclists have a race.
This graph shows how far each one
goes in 1 second, 2 seconds, etc.

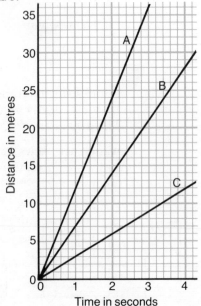

(a) Which cyclist went furthest in
1 second?

(b) Which cyclist is slowest?

(c) How far did B go in 1 second?

(d) What is B's speed?

(e) What is A's speed?

(f) What is C's speed?

(g) How far apart are A and C
3 seconds from the start?

B6 A girl runs at 7 m/s for 3 seconds.
Then she changes speed and walks at 4 m/s for 5 seconds.

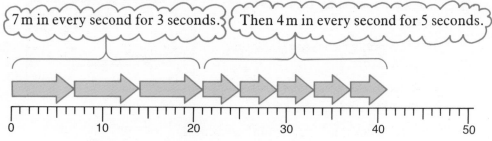

7 m in every second for 3 seconds. Then 4 m in every second for 5 seconds.

(a) Copy and complete this table.

Time in seconds	0	1	2	3	4	5	6	7	8
Distance in metres									

(b) Draw axes on graph paper, with time across and distance up.
Draw the graph.

B7 A car travels at 20 m/s for 4 seconds, then at 10 m/s for 6 seconds.

(a) Copy and complete this table.

Time in seconds	0	1	2	3	4	5	6	7	8	9	10
Distance in metres	0	20				90					

(b) Draw a graph, with time across and distance up.

B8 A sports car, travelling at 30 m/s, overtakes an old banger,
travelling at 7 m/s.

(a) How far does the sports car go in the next 15 seconds?
(b) How far does the banger go in 15 seconds?
(c) How far apart are the two cars 15 seconds after overtaking?
(d) How far apart are they 1 minute after overtaking?

B9 Here is a graph for a runner.

Which of these sentences fits the
graph?

A   He went quite slowly at first,
then speeded up and then speeded
up again.

B   He went quite fast at first,
then slowed down, then speeded up.

C   He went quite fast at first,
then slowed down, then slowed
down again.

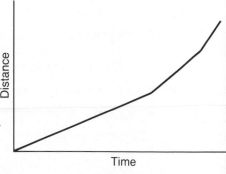

c Volume

C1 This model is made from centimetre cubes.

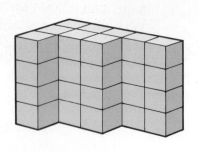

    (a) How many cubes are there in each layer?

    (b) What is the volume of the model in cubic cm?

C2 What is the volume of each of these models?

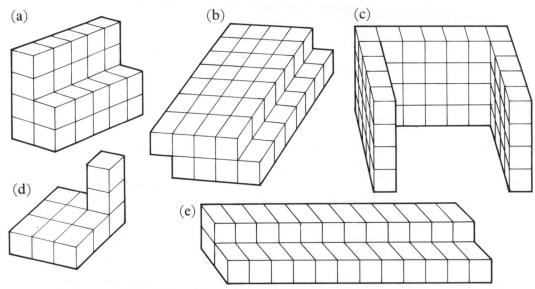

(a)   (b)   (c)

(d)   (e)

C3 One of the models in question C2 is **not** a prism. Which one is it?

C4 Which of these are prisms?

    (a)   (b)   (c)   (d)

C5 Work out   (i) the area of the cross-section
             (ii) the volume
    of each of these prisms.

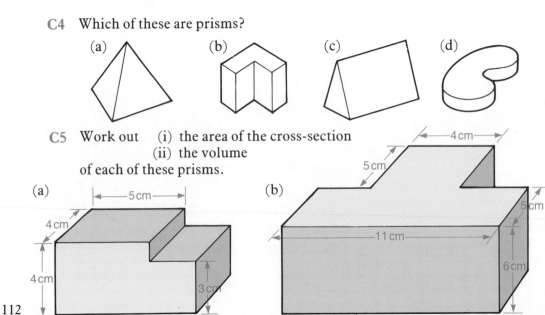

(a)   5 cm   (b)   4 cm

4 cm   5 cm

4 cm   3 cm   11 cm   5 cm

8 cm   6 cm

1 Area (1)

E1.1 (a) Calculate the area of the coloured right-angled triangle.

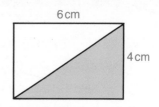

Calculate the area of each of these right-angled triangles.

(b)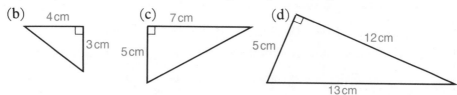

(c)

(d)

E1.2 (a) Write down the lengths of AB and AD, and calculate the area of the rectangle ABCD.

(b) Calculate the area of each of the four right-angled triangles in the diagram, and add up the four areas.

(c) Calculate the area of the coloured shape.

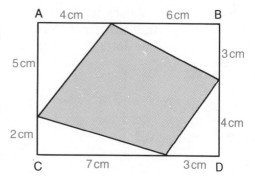

E1.3 Calculate the area of each coloured shape below. All lengths are marked in centimetres.

(a)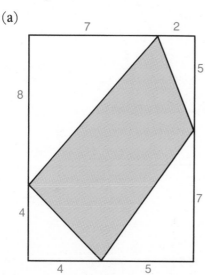

(b)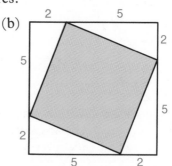

(c)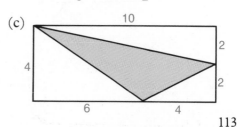

113

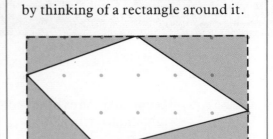

| You can find the area of this shape . . . | by thinking of a rectangle around it. |

E1.4 The shape above is drawn on 1 cm square spotty paper.

(a) Calculate the area of the dotted rectangle.

(b) Calculate the total area of the four shaded right-angled triangles.

(c) Calculate the area of the unshaded shape.

E1.5 Calculate the area of each of these shapes.
Draw them on spotty paper if you want to.
(The dotted lines are drawn on the first one, to help you.)

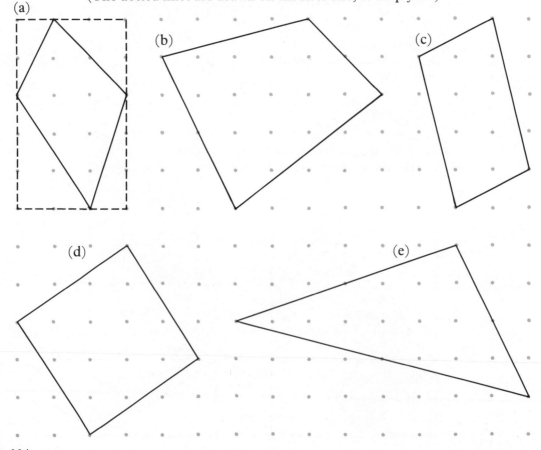

(a)

(b)

(c)

(d)

(e)

2 Patterns (1)

Use this standard set of figures for questions E2.1 and E2.2.

0 1 2 3 4 5 6 7 8 9

E2.1   This three-figure number has a two-fold rotation centre:

6 ǂ 9

This three-figure number has a 2-fold rotation centre and two lines of reflection symmetry.

-8-φ-8-

What other three-figure numbers have

(a) a 2-fold rotation centre, but no reflection symmetry

(b) a 2-fold rotation centre, and lines of reflection symmetry

E2.2   One way of writing dates is to use three numbers separated by dashes.

For example, 24 – 5 – 76 means '24th May 1976'.

Some dates have a 2-fold rotation centre, for example:

19 - 8 - 61

What other dates can you find which have a 2-fold rotation centre? (Some may have reflection symmetry as well.)

E2.3   Copy this diagram.

Colour **two** more squares so that the design has a 4-fold rotation centre.

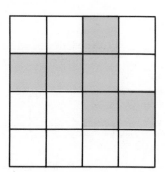

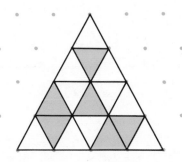

E2.4   Copy this diagram.

Colour one more triangle so that the design has a 3-fold rotation centre.

5 Decimals

E5.1 This scale is marked in **fifths**.

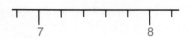

You can imagine the tenths marks
which are in between the fifths marks.

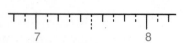

Write down the numbers marked below. ((a) is **not** 5·2!)

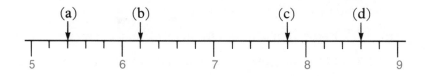

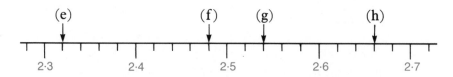

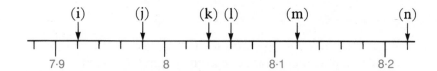

E5.2 These scales are marked in different ways.
Write down the numbers which the arrows point to.

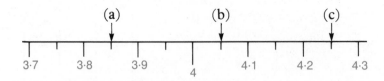

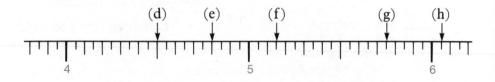

6 Multiplication

'Forensic science' is the name given to scientific methods used by the police to investigate crime.

When human bones are found, a forensic scientist can calculate quite accurately the height of the person whose bones they were.

If a thigh bone (called the **femur**) is found, these rules are used to work out the person's height. All measurements are in centimetres.

Males
Height = (length of femur × 2·238) + 69·089

Females
Height = (length of femur × 2·317) + 61·412

E6.1 A male femur of length 51·3 cm has been found. Calculate the owner's height. Round off the height to the nearest whole centimetre.

E6.2 A female femur of length 35·7 cm has been found. Calculate the woman's height to the nearest centimetre.

These are the rules for calculating the height from other measurements.

Bone	Males	Females
Tibia	Height = (length × 2·392) + 81·688	Height = (length × 2·533) + 72·572
Humerus	Height = (length × 2·970) + 73·570	Height = (length × 3·144) + 64·977
Radius	Height = (length × 3·650) + 80·405	Height = (length × 3·876) + 73·502

E6.3 Work out the heights, to the nearest cm, of the people who owned these bones.
(a) A female humerus of length 32·9 cm
(b) A male tibia of length 40·2 cm
(c) A male radius of length 33·0 cm
(d) A female tibia of length 37·9 cm

E6.4 A detective has found these two female bones.

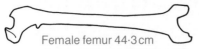
Female femur 44·3 cm

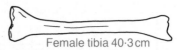
Female tibia 40·3 cm

He wants to know if they could have belonged to the same person. So he calculates the height of the owner of each bone.
(a) Calculate the height of the owner of the femur.
(b) Calculate the height of the owner of the tibia.
(c) Could the bones be from the same person?

8 Division

These problems require multiplication and division.

E8.1 Helical Products sell bolts in boxes containing 144 bolts.
144 bolts weigh 4·9 kg.

(a) What does one bolt weigh? Give the weight in kg, to 3 d.p.

(b) Helical Products decide to sell the bolts in boxes of 100.
What will 100 bolts weigh? Give the weight in kg, to 1 d.p.

E8.2 A group of 34 people want to go to Brighton for the day.
If they go by train, the fare is £2·35 each.
If they hire a coach, it would cost £73 altogether.

(a) How much will each person have to pay if the group hires a coach? (Round off your answer to the nearest penny.)

(b) Is the coach cheaper than the train?

(c) If there were only 30 people in the group, it would still cost £73 to hire a coach.
Would it be cheaper for 30 people to hire a coach or to go by train?
What is the difference in the cost per person?

E8.3

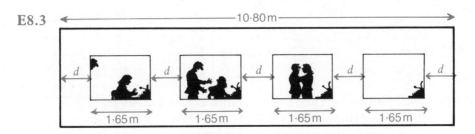

These four pictures are mounted on the wall of an art gallery. The distances marked d are all equal.

Calculate d. Show your method.

E8.4

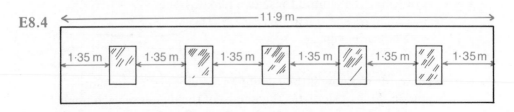

This wall is 11·9 m long. Every window has the same width.
Calculate the width of each window.

E8.5 Petrol in France cost 4·39 francs per litre (in 1984).
A gallon is approximately equal to 4·55 litres.
1 French franc was worth 8·7 pence (in 1984).

Calculate the cost in pence of a gallon of petrol in France,
to the nearest penny.

E8.6 Two shops both sell Spanish onions of the same quality.
Shop A sells them for 38p per kilogram.
Shop B sells them in 3 lb packs. A 3 lb pack costs 49p.

(a) 1 lb is equal to 0·454 kg.
What is the weight in kilograms of a 3 lb pack?

(b) In which shop are the onions cheaper? Give the
reason for your answer.

E8.7 Six photographs have to be fixed to an exhibition stand.
The stand is 200 cm by 120 cm, and it may be
this way up, 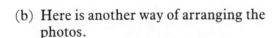 or this way up.

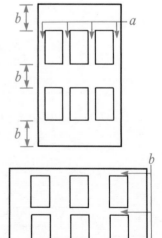

Each photo is 45 cm by 25 cm and must
be this way up.

(a) Here is one way of arranging the six photos.

If the gaps marked *a* are all equal,
and those marked *b* are all equal,
calculate *a* and *b*, to the nearest 0·1 cm.

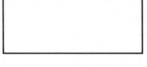

(b) Here is another way of arranging the
photos.

Calculate *a* and *b* in this case, to the
nearest 0·1 cm.

(c) Sketch another way of arranging the
photos, with equal spacing across
and equal spacing up.

Calculate the width of the gaps in your arrangement, to the
nearest 0·1 cm.

9 Flow charts

E9.1 Each shape on the right is made up of 5 squares.

Some of the shapes can be cut out and folded to make a box without a lid.

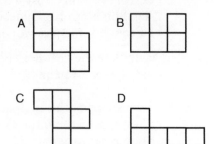

A boy drew this flow chart. He says it will tell you whether or not each shape will make a box without a lid.

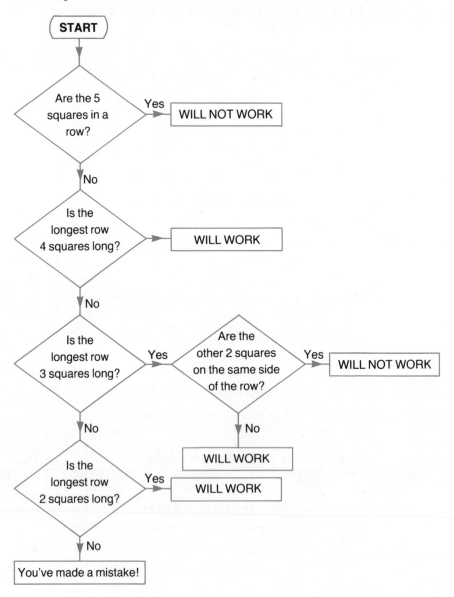

(a) Use the flow chart with each of the shapes A to D.
Does the flow chart give the correct answer for each shape?

Check by drawing the shapes on squared paper, cutting them out and folding them.

(b) What other shapes can you make by joining 5 equal squares together edge to edge? (Joining only at corners is not allowed. So this, for example, is not allowed: 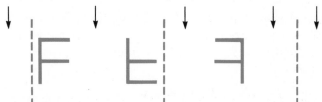)

Can you find any shapes for which the flow chart gives the wrong answer?

10 Patterns (2)

E10.1 This is part of a repeating pattern, but some pictures are missing. The arrows show where the missing pictures go. The dotted lines are lines of reflection symmetry.

Copy the pattern and draw the missing pictures.

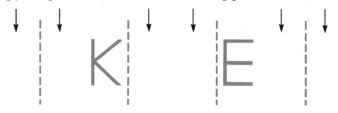

E10.2 Do the same as before for this pattern.

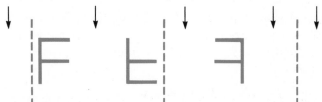

E10.3 Draw this pattern on squared paper and mark its 2-fold rotation centres.

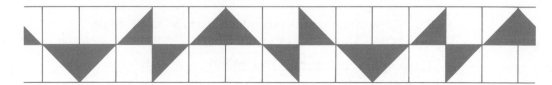

12 Formulas and graphs

E12.1 Pam's school has a Spring Fair and she is asked to get some leaflets printed to advertise it. She knows a photocopying shop which charges 5p a copy.

(a) Copy this table and complete it.

Number of copies	0	200	400	600	800	1000
Cost in £	0					

(b) Draw axes on graph paper. Use the scales shown here.

Plot the points from your table and draw the graph.

The graph is a straight line. Label the line 'Photocopying'.

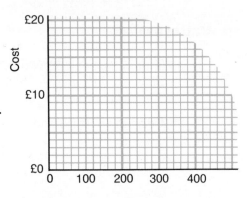

(c) Pam goes to a printer to find out how much it would cost to have the leaflets printed.

The printer charges £35 for making the 'plate' from which copies are printed. Then he charges 50p per 100 copies. (So the total cost of, say, 600 copies is £35 plus 6 × 50p, which is £38.)

Copy this table and complete it.

Number of copies	0	200	400	600	800	1000
Cost in £	35					

(d) Plot the points from the second table **on the same graph as the first**. Draw the graph and label it 'Printing'.

(e) The graphs show that for small numbers of copies it is cheaper to photocopy, but for large numbers it is cheaper to print. Use the graphs to find the number of copies for which the two methods cost the same.

E12.2 If $a = 5$, $b = 4$ and $c = 3$, work out the value of

(a) $2a + b$ (b) $4b - 3a$ (c) $a + \dfrac{b}{2}$ (d) $\dfrac{12}{c} - b$

(e) $\dfrac{8a}{b}$ (f) $a + 2b + 5c$ (g) $b - \dfrac{a}{2}$ (h) $\dfrac{2c}{b}$

E12.3 A factory makes toy cars out of metal. Every now and then they bring out a new model. The price they charge for a car depends on how many they make. The more they make, the cheaper the cars are.

If they think a new model will be very popular with children, they make a large number and they can then charge a low price.

If they think a new model·will appeal to fewer children, they do not make so many and the price has to be higher.

There is a formula connecting the price with the number made. It is

$$p = 30 + \frac{24\,000}{n}.$$

p is the price of a car in pence.
n is the number made.

(a) Calculate p when n is 1000, 2000, 3000, and so on up to 6000, and write the results in a table.

n (number of cars made)	1000	2000	3000	4000	5000	6000
p (price of one car, in pence)	54					

(b) Draw a graph with n across and p up.

Use the scales shown here.

The graph is a **curve**, not a straight line.

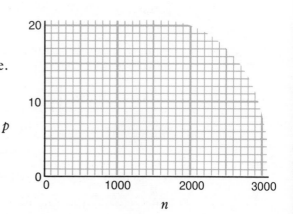

(c) Use the graph to find the number of cars the factory should make if the selling price is to be 40p per car.

123

M Miscellaneous

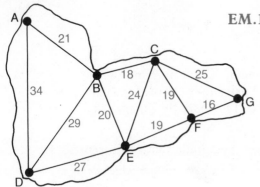

EM.1 This is a road map of an island.
A, B, C, D, E, F and G are seven towns.

The numbers show distances in miles.

There is a SupaValue shop in each of the seven towns.

(a) The seven managers of the shops need to meet to discuss
   price rises. The meeting can be held at either B, C, E or F.

   (i) If all the managers travel to B, what is the total of all
   their travelling distances?

   (ii) Calculate the total travelling distance for each of the
   other possible meeting places C, E and F.

   (iii) Which of the four meeting places should the managers choose
   if they want the total travelling distance to be as small
   as possible?

(b) The warehouse which supplies all the shops is at B.
   A delivery van starts from B and visits every shop before
   returning to B. What is the shortest route for it to take?
   (Give the order in which the van visits the other shops.)

(c) As in (b), but this time the van also has to pick up a box at A and
   deliver it to E, and to pick up a box at G to deliver to F.

EM.2

This pattern continues downwards.

(a) Work out the numbers
   which will go here.

   Explain how you do it.

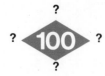

(b) Work out the numbers at the four
   corners of diamond number 573.

124

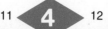